The ECG in practice

For Churchill Livingstone

Publisher: Laurence Hunter
Project Manager: Ninette Premdas
Copy Editor: Alison Gale
Project Controller: Kay Hunston
Design: Erik Bigland

The ECG
in practice

John R. Hampton DM MA DPhil FRCP FFPM FESC
Professor of Cardiology
University of Nottingham
Nottingham
UK

THIRD EDITION

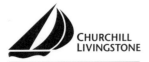

CHURCHILL
LIVINGSTONE

EDINBURGH LONDON NEW YORK PHILADELPHIA
SYDNEY TORONTO 1997

CHURCHILL LIVINGSTONE
A Medical Division of Harcourt Brace and Company Limited

© Harcourt Brace and Company Limited

⚓ is a registered trademark of Harcourt Brace and Company Limited

The right of Professor J. R. Hampton to be identified as author of this
Work has been asserted by him in accordance with the Copyright, Designs
and Patents Act 1988.

First edition 1986
Second edition 1992
Third edition 1997
   Reprinted 1998

ISBN 0 443 056803

British Library of Cataloguing in Publication Data
A catalogue record for this book is available from the British Library.

Library of Congress Cataloging in Publication Data
A catalog record for this book is available from the Library of Congress.

Medical knowledge is constantly changing. As new information becomes
available, changes in treatment, procedures, equipment and the use of
drugs become necessary. The author and the publishers have, as far as it
is possible, taken care to ensure that the information given in this text is
accurate and up to date. However, readers are strongly advised to confirm
that the information, especially with regard to drug usage, complies with
current legislation and standards of practice.

Printed in China
GCC/02

Contents

Preface

This book assumes that the reader has the level of knowledge about the ECG that is contained in *The ECG made easy*, to which this is a companion volume. The principal tenets of *The ECG made easy* are that the ECG is easy to understand and that its abnormalities are perfectly logical. The normal ECG and typical examples of abnormal ECGs are indeed easy to interpret. However, ECG interpretation sometimes appears more difficult than it really is because of the variations that can occur, in the normal record and in the abnormal ECGs that are associated with various diseases. This book therefore looks beyond typical ECGs, and attempts to describe the variations that are seen in health and in disease. It is intended for senior medical students, specialist nurses, junior hospital doctors and indeed for anyone who makes – or intends to make – frequent use of the ECG in the management of patients.

The second purpose of this book is to demonstrate that an ECG should always be interpreted in the light of information about the individual from whom it was recorded. Recording and interpreting the ECG are, in fact, extensions of taking the clinical history and performing a physical examination. The ECG is not an end in itself but is part of the process of diagnosis and management of an individual patient, so this book approaches the ECG from the standpoint of the different clinical symptoms of cardiovascular disease. To emphasize the secondary role of the ECG in diagnosis, each chapter begins with a brief consideration of how the history and physical examination can be used to make, or at least suspect, a diagnosis – so enabling the use of the ECG in the most intelligent and profitable way.

There is no point in recording an ECG unless you know what to do with the result, so at the end of each chapter there is a brief section outlining the action that should follow the identification of ECG abnormalities, followed by one or two ECG records to provide examples of ECG interpretation.

One of the fascinating things about the ECG is the amount of information it provides about the normal and pathological physiology of the heart. Knowing about this is by no means essential for making use of the ECG, but certainly helps in its understanding. Nevertheless, many people will make good use of the ECG without ever wanting to know about its physiological basis, the description of which is placed in Chapter 6.

I am extremely grateful to Mr G. Lyth for preparing the illustrations, to Professor Sheila Gardner for advice, and to Mrs Alison Gale for help with the manuscript.

Nottingham, 1997   J. R. H.

Introduction

WHAT TO EXPECT OF THE ECG

The ECG is an invaluable tool for the investigation and management of people with cardiovascular problems – but do not expect too much from it. Like everything else in medicine, the ECG is not infallible: abnormal ECGs may not be clinically important, and normal ECGs can conceal severe cardiac disease.

The most important thing to remember when considering the ECG is that it provides a picture only of the electrical activity within the heart. It gives no direct information about the efficiency of the heart as a pump, nor about the state of the valves, coronary arteries, or heart muscle – though it is quite often possible to infer things about structure and function from the electrical picture. The ECG is most useful, and indeed it is essential, for the diagnosis and management of electrical cardiac problems (conduction defects and arrhythmias), but its limitations in other circumstances must be recognized.

An ECG is usually recorded in one of four sets of circumstances:

- people without apparent cardiovascular problems (as part of either 'health screening' or pre-operative assessment)
- people complaining of palpitations or attacks of dizziness (when an arrhythmia is suspected)
- people with chest pain (when there is usually a possibility of cardiac ischaemia)
- people with breathlessness (when there may be difficulty in distinguishing between heart failure, lung disease, and a simple lack of physical fitness).

This book discusses the use of the ECG in these different circumstances, with a chapter devoted to each.

In healthy people, or those due for non-cardiovascular surgery, the finding of a normal ECG is reassuring. However, it is important to remember that the ECG can remain normal despite severe narrowing of all three main coronary arteries, so a normal ECG in itself does not guarantee longevity, nor does it even indicate fitness for general anaesthesia. Conversely, finding an abnormal ECG in the absence of apparent cardiovascular problems does not necessarily matter. There is a range of normality, and undoubted abnormalities such as bundle branch block, do not necessarily indicate significant cardiac problems. It is the patient's clinical state that really matters, and the ECG is only one part of its assessment.

When a patient complains of palpitations or dizziness, an ECG will suggest a diagnosis if it is recorded when the patient has symptoms. Dizziness with a normal ECG at the time is not due to a cardiac problem; palpitations (an awareness of the heartbeat) may or may not be due to an arrhythmia, and an ECG recorded during an attack will help in deciding the cause. In the nature of things, however, patients seldom have their symptoms while an ECG is being recorded, and the ECG record then simply becomes one more piece of evidence to add to the history and examination before making the diagnosis.

In a patient with chest pain, the ECG can be diagnostic or downright misleading. The proper use of thrombolytics in acute myocardial infarction depends on the presence of characteristic ECG changes, but the ECG can remain normal for several hours after a coronary occlusion. Following an infarction, the ECG can remain abnormal even though the patient has made a full recovery, or can return to normal. In angina, the ECG will usually become abnormal during an attack of pain, but this is by no means always the case. Again, it is the total clinical picture of history, examination and ECG that matters.

The patient who is breathless because of heart failure is unlikely to have a totally normal ECG, but there needs to be quite severe lung disease before the ECG becomes abnormal. A proper history and examination are more helpful than the ECG in reaching a diagnosis, but at least a normal ECG in a breathless patient indicates that more detailed cardiac investigation, such as echocardiography, is unlikely to be helpful.

Finally, the ECG may give clues to non-cardiac problems which are sometimes unexpected, and it is essential to remember that the ECG can be affected by drugs, electrolytic abnormalities, and malignancy.

These limitations should not be seen as making the ECG unimportant and unreliable, but they do place it in perspective. The ECG can only be a part of patient assessment, and it must take its proper place – often a secondary place – in relation to the history and examination. The ECG is perhaps best thought of as a natural progression beyond the stethoscope; it is simply the next stage of the examination.

HOW TO REPORT AN ECG

An ECG can be described in isolation, but a sensible report can only be given if the reason for recording it is known.

The standard description of an ECG should include the rhythm; the heart rate; a comment on conduction both into and within the ventricles; and comments on the shapes of the QRS complexes, the ST segments, and the T waves. Ideally it should be possible to conclude that the trace is either normal or abnormal, but it must be accepted that many records cannot easily be classified so, and a category of 'probably within normal limits' is realistic.

When the reason for recording the ECG is known, a full report can be given, including clinical interpretation and suggestions for further investigation and management. As with any medical investigation, it is important to separate the description, which is factual, and the interpretation, which to some extent depends on opinion.

The presentation of ECG records

There is a variety of ways in which the paper record of an ECG can be presented, and since rapid ECG interpretation is a matter of pattern recognition, different formats can cause confusion. In the United Kingdom, North America, and most of the rest of the world, the speed of the paper is always 25 mm/s. In some

European countries, however, a speed of 50 mm/s is used and the visual appearance of the ECG is quite different.

For the interpretation of a rhythm, any single lead that shows it clearly will do, but frequently it is necessary to inspect all 12 leads to see which demonstrates the rhythm most clearly. In this book, single 'rhythm strips' are used when only a rhythm is being discussed, and the reader must assume that the clearest of the 12 leads has been selected.

12-lead ECGs are now usually displayed in horizontal format on A4 paper, which presents a problem for reproduction in a book such as this. Sometimes leads I, II and III are presented vertically on the left-hand side of the sheet; then VR, VL and VF; then V_1, V_2 and V_3; and finally V_4, V_5 and V_6 on the right-hand side. Sometimes the six limb leads are shown in a vertical sequence on the left-hand side of the sheet, opposite the six chest leads. The former presentation has been used in this book. A few full records (inevitably somewhat reduced) are included to aid the development of pattern recognition, but in general 12 leads are shown as one complex from each lead, arranged in the standard way – this has allowed a 12-lead record to be presented on a single vertical page.

CHAPTER 1

The ECG in healthy people

THE RANGE OF NORMALITY IN THE ECG

For the purposes of this chapter we shall assume that the subject from whom the ECG was recorded is asymptomatic, and that physical examination has revealed no abnormalities. We need to consider the range of normality of the ECG, but of course we cannot escape from the fact that not all disease causes symptoms or abnormal physical signs, and a subject who appears healthy may not be so. In particular, individuals who present for 'screening' may well have symptoms about which they have not consulted a doctor, so it cannot be assumed that an ECG obtained through a screening programme has come from a healthy subject.

The range of normality in the ECG is therefore debatable – we have first to consider the variations in the ECG that we can expect to find in completely healthy people, and then we can think about the significance of abnormalities.

ACCEPTABLE VARIATIONS IN THE NORMAL ECG

The normal cardiac rhythm

Sinus rhythm is the only normal sustained rhythm. In young people the R–R interval is reduced (that is, the heart rate is increased) during inspiration, and this is called sinus arrhythmia. When sinus arrhythmia is marked, it may mimic an atrial arrhythmia. However, in sinus arrhythmia each P–QRS–T complex is normal, and it is only the interval between them that changes.

SINUS ARRHYTHMIA

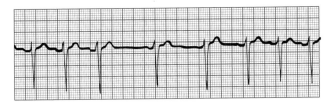

Note: Marked variation in R–R interval
         Constant PR interval
         Constant shape of P wave and QRS complex.

Sinus arrhythmia becomes less marked with increasing age of the subject, and is lost in conditions such as diabetic autonomic neuropathy, in both situations because vagus nerve function is impaired.

Occasionally, sinus arrhythmia can cause such a long R–R interval that an escape beat occurs.

Extrasystoles

Supraventricular extrasystoles, either atrial or junctional (AV nodal) commonly occur in normal people and are of no significance.

SUPRAVENTRICULAR EXTRASYSTOLES

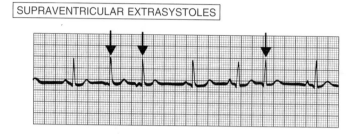

Note: In supraventricular extrasystoles the QRS complexes and T waves are the same as in the sinus beats
Atrial extrasystoles have an abnormal P wave
Junctional extrasystoles have no P wave.

Ventricular extrasystoles are also commonly seen in normal ECGs. Their significance will be discussed in Chapter 2.

VENTRICULAR EXTRASYSTOLES

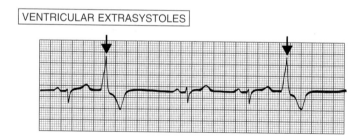

Note: The ventricular extrasystoles are identified by the absence of a P wave, and the abnormal QRS complex and T wave.

The P wave

In sinus rhythm, the P wave is normally upright in all leads except
VR. When the QRS complex is predominantly downward in VL,
the P wave may also be inverted.

NORMAL ECG

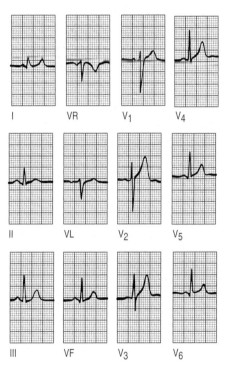

I   VR V_1 V_4

II   VL V_2 V_5

III   VF V_3 V_6

Note: In both VR and VL the P wave is inverted, and the QRS
complex is predominantly downward.

In patients with dextrocardia, the P wave is inverted in lead I – although in practice this pattern is more often seen when the limb electrodes have been wrongly attached.

DEXTROCARDIA

Note: In dextrocardia the
P wave is inverted
in lead I
The chest leads
V_1–V_6 show right
ventricular
complexes
Electrodes placed
on the right side
of the chest, in
positions
corresponding
to those of the
normal V leads
on the left side,
show that the left
ventricle underlies
the V_6 position on
the right side of
the chest (V_6R).

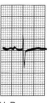

V_4R

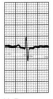

V_5R

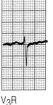

V_3R

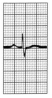

V_6R

The PR interval

In sinus rhythm, the PR interval is constant and the normal range is 120–220 ms (3–5 small squares of ECG paper).

NORMAL ECG

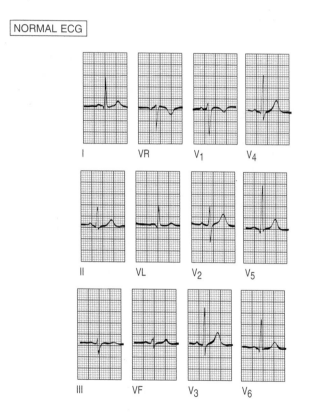

I   VR V_1 V_4

II   VL V_2 V_5

III   VF V_3 V_6

Note: Sinus rhythm: the PR interval is constant in all leads, at 160 ms.

A PR interval of less than 120 ms suggests pre-excitation, and a PR interval longer than 220 ms is due to first degree block: these will be discussed further in Chapter 2.

The QRS complex

The cardiac axis

There is a fairly wide range of normality in the direction of the cardiac axis. In most people the QRS complex is tallest in lead II, but in leads I and III the QRS is also predominantly upright (i.e. the R wave is greater than the S wave).

NORMAL ECG

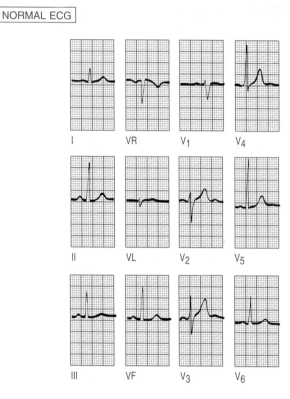

| I | VR | V₁ | V₄ |

| II | VL | V₂ | V₅ |

| III | VF | V₃ | V₆ |

Note: With a normal cardiac axis the QRS complex is predominantly upright in leads I, II and III, but is tallest in lead II.

The cardiac axis is still normal when the R wave and the S wave are equal in lead I: this pattern is common in tall subjects.

NORMAL ECG

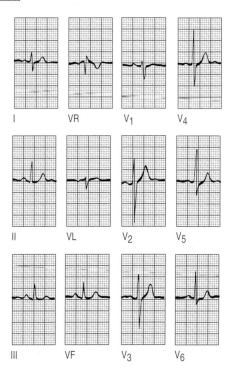

I VR V₁ V₄

II VL V₂ V₅

III VF V₃ V₆

Note: The record shows the limit of normality of the cardiac axis
The R and S waves are equal in lead I.

When the S wave is greater than the R wave in lead I, right axis deviation is present (see Ch. 4).

It is common for the S wave to be greater than the R wave in lead III, and the cardiac axis can still be considered normal when the S wave equals the R wave in lead II. This combination of patterns in leads II and III is common in fat people and during pregnancy.

NORMAL ECG

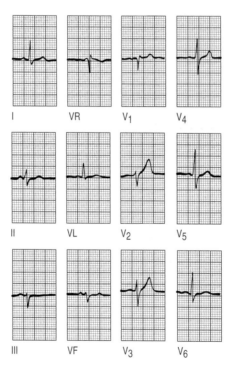

Note: This record shows the limit of normality of the cardiac axis
The S wave is greater than the R wave in lead III
The S wave equals the R wave in lead II.

When the depth of the S wave exceeds the height of the R wave in lead II, left axis deviation is present (see Chs 2 and 6).

The size of R and S waves in the chest leads

In lead V_1 there should be a small R wave and a deep S wave, and the balance between the two should change progressively from V_1–V_6. In V_6 there should be a tall R wave and no S wave.

Loss of this normal 'progression' of the R wave, with a sudden increase in its height in V_5 or V_6, can indicate an old anterior infarction.

NORMAL ECG

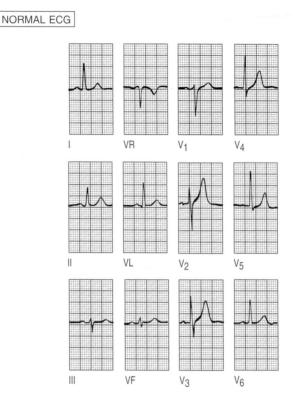

I   VR V_1 V_4

II   VL V_2 V_5

III   VF V_3 V_6

Note: This record shows normal QRS complexes in the V leads. There is a progressive change of pattern from V_1–V_6, with the R and S waves equal in V_3.

Very occasionally the ECG of a totally normal subject will show a 'dominant R wave' (that is, the height of the R wave exceeds the depth of the S wave) in V_1.

NORMAL ECG

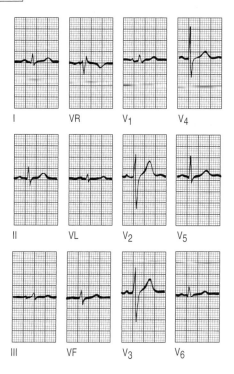

Note: In V_1 the height of the R wave exceeds the depth of the S wave.

However, the presence of a dominant R wave in V_1 is usually due either to a true posterior infarction or to right ventricular hypertrophy (see Chs 3 and 4 respectively).

Although the balance between the height of the R wave and the depth of the S wave is significant for identifying the direction of the cardiac axis and for the identification of right ventricular hypertrophy, the absolute height of the R wave provides little useful information. It is, of course, important that the ECG is properly calibrated with 1 mV causing 1 cm of vertical deflection on the ECG. The limits for the size of the R and S waves in normal subjects are sometimes set at 25 mm for the R wave in V_5 or V_6, or for the S wave in V_1 or V_2. In addition, the sum of the R wave in V_5 or V_6 and the S wave in V_1 or V_2 is supposed to be less than 35 mm. However, R waves taller than 25 mm are commonly seen in V_5–V_6 in fit and thin young people, and are perfectly normal.

NORMAL ECG

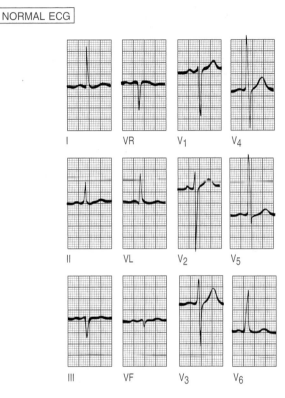

I   VR   V₁   V₄

II   VL   V₂   V₅

III   VF   V₃   V₆

Note: Normal ECG from a young man
R wave in lead V_5 is 28 mm high, and S wave in V_2 is
28 mm deep.

The width of the QRS complex

The QRS complex should be less than 3 mm across (i.e. of less than 120 ms duration) in all leads. If it is wider than this, then either the ventricles have been depolarized from a ventricular rather than a supraventricular focus (i.e. a ventricular rhythm is present), or there is an abnormality of conduction within the ventricles. The latter is most commonly due to bundle branch block.

An RSR[1] pattern in V_1, resembling that of right bundle branch block but with a narrow QRS complex, is sometimes called 'partial right bundle branch block', and is a normal variant.

NORMAL ECG

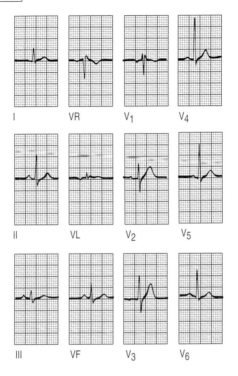

I	VR	V₁	V₄
II	VL	V₂	V₅
III	VF	V₃	V₆

Note: Partial right bundle branch block
RSR^1 complex in V$_1$, with QRS duration 120 ms.

Q waves

The normal depolarization of the interventricular septum from left to right to causes a small 'septal' Q wave in any of leads II, VL or V_5–V_6. Septal Q waves are less than 2 mm deep and less than 1 mm across.

NORMAL ECG

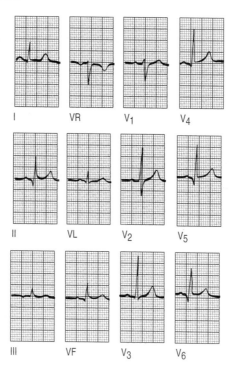

Note: Normal depolarization of the septum causes small Q waves in leads II, V_5 and V_6.

A small Q wave is also common in lead III; when normal, such a Q wave is always narrow but can occasionally be more than 2 mm deep. These Q waves usually disappear during deep inspiration, due to movement of the heart.

NORMAL ECG

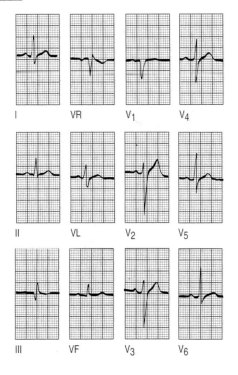

(continued on next page)

Deep inspiration

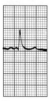

III

Note: Normal Q wave in lead III
No Q wave in lead VF
Q wave in lead III disappears on inspiration.

When a Q wave is present in lead VF as well as in lead III, an inferior infarction is likely (see Ch. 3).

The ST segment

The ST segment (the part of the ECG between the S wave and the T wave) should be horizontal and 'isoelectric', which means that it should be at the same level on the paper as the baseline of the record between the end of the T wave and the next P wave.

NORMAL ECG

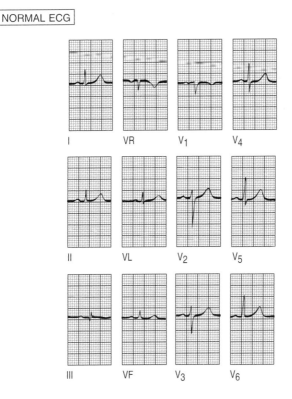

I	VR	V₁	V₄
II	VL	V₂	V₅
III	VF	V₃	V₆

Note: In all leads the ST segment is isoelectric.

An elevation of the ST segment is the hallmark of an acute myocardial infarction, and depression of the ST segment can indicate ischaemia or the effect of digitalis. However, it is perfectly normal for the ST segment to be elevated following an S wave in leads V_2–V_5; this is sometimes called a 'high take-off ST segment'.

NORMAL ECG

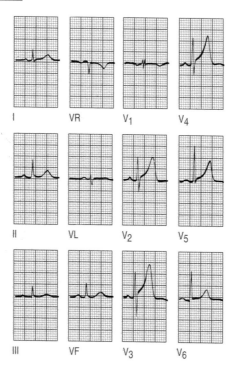

| I | VR | V_1 | V_4 |

| II | VL | V_2 | V_5 |

| III | VF | V_3 | V_6 |

Note: In leads V_2–V_5 the ST segment is elevated following an S wave.

Depression of the ST segment is common in normal people and especially in pregnancy, but in such 'non-specific' depression the ST segment is not more than 2 mm below the baseline, and it is either convex downward, or slopes upwards from the S wave to the T wave. ST segment depression of more than 2 mm usually indicates ischaemia (see Ch. 3).

The T wave

In normal ECGs the T wave is always inverted in VR, but is usually upright in all the other leads.

NORMAL ECG

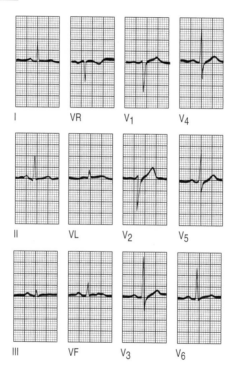

Note: T wave is inverted in VR but is upright in all other leads.

The T wave is often inverted in lead III but becomes more upright on inspiration (see p. 26 above). The T wave is also often inverted in V_1.

NORMAL ECG

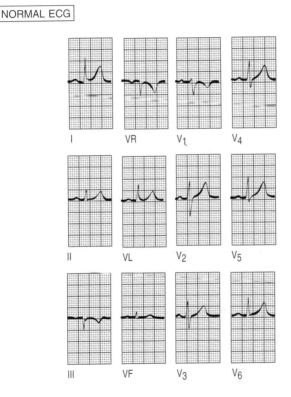

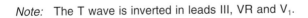

Note: The T wave is inverted in leads III, VR and V_1.

T wave inversion in V_2–V_3 as well as in V_1 occurs in right ventricular hypertrophy, but it can be a normal variant, particularly in black people.

NORMAL ECG (BLACK WOMAN)

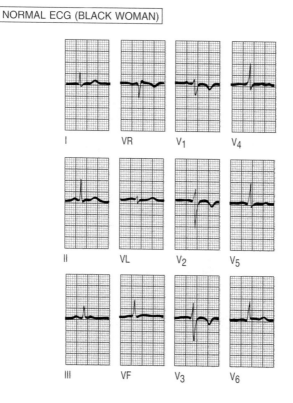

I   VR V_1 V_4

II   VL V_2 V_5

III   VF V_3 V_6

Note: ECG from a black person
The T wave is inverted in V_1–V_3.

Generalized flattening of the T waves with a normal QT interval is best described as 'non-specific'.

NORMAL ECG

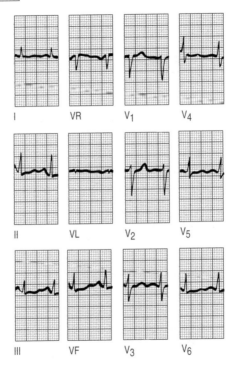

Note: The T waves show non-specific flattening in several leads.

Peaked T waves are characteristic of hyperkalaemia, but they are also common in healthy people.

NORMAL ECG

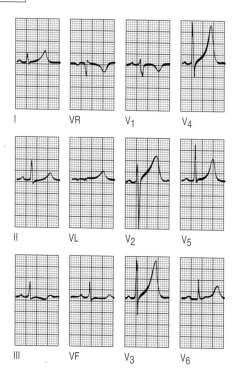

I   VR   V₁   V₄

II   VL   V₂   V₅

III   VF   V₃   V₆

Note: Peaked T waves in V_2–V_4.

The T wave is the most variable part of the ECG, both between individuals and in the same individual at different times. It may become inverted in some leads simply by the hyperventilation associated with anxiety.

An extra hump on the end of the T wave, a 'U' wave, is characteristic of hypokalaemia, but U waves are commonly seen in the anterior chest leads of normal ECGs. They are thought to be due to repolarization of the papillary muscles.

NORMAL ECG

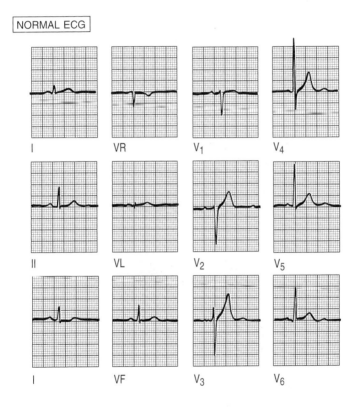

Note: Prominent U waves in V_3–V_5.

The QT interval

The QT interval (Q wave to the end of the T wave) varies with the heart rate, gender and time of day. There are several different ways of correcting for heart rate, but the simplest is by Bazett's formula, in which QT_c is the corrected length of the QT interval:

$$QT_c = \frac{QT}{\sqrt{R–R \text{ interval}}}$$

It is, however, uncertain whether QT_c has any greater clinical significance than the uncorrected QT interval. The normal QT interval is 350–430 ms, and whatever the rate, a QT interval of greater than 440 ms is probably pathological.

THE ECG IN ATHLETES

Most of the normal variations discussed above are common in athletes. Below are listed some of the ECG features that might be considered abnormal in non-athletic subjects, but normal in athletes.

Variations in rhythm:
- Sinus bradycardia
- Marked sinus arrhythmia
- Junctional rhythm
- 'Wandering' atrial pacemaker
- First degree block
- Wenckebach block.

Variations in ECG pattern:
- Tall P waves
- Tall R waves and deep S waves
- Prominent septal Q waves
- Counter-clockwise rotation
- Slight ST segment elevation
- Tall symmetrical T waves
- T wave inversion, especially in lateral leads
- Biphasic T waves
- Prominent U waves.

THE ECG IN CHILDREN

The normal heart rate in the first year of life is 140–160 per minute, falling slowly to about 80 per minute by puberty. Sinus arrhythmia is usually quite marked in children.

At birth, the muscle of the right ventricle is as thick as that of the left ventricle and the ECG of a normal child in the first year of life has a pattern that would indicate right ventricular hypertrophy in an adult.

NORMAL ECG: AT BIRTH

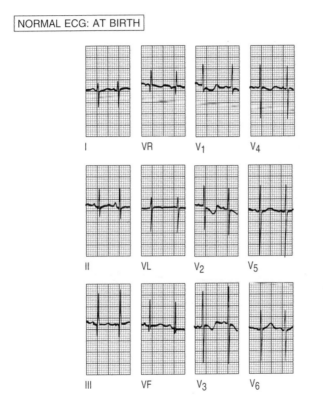

Note: Sinus rhythm, 160 per minute
Right axis deviation
Dominant R waves in V_1
Deep S waves in V_5 and V_6
Inverted T waves in V_1–V_4.

These features gradually disappear.

NORMAL ECG: AGE 1 YEAR

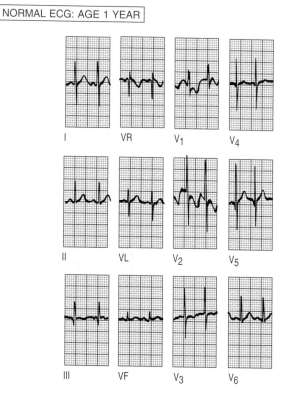

Note: Sinus rhythm, 150 per minute
Right axis deviation
Dominant R waves in V_1
Inverted T waves in V_1–V_3.

NORMAL ECG: AGE 2 YEARS

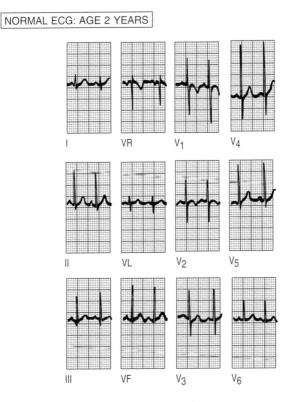

I   VR   V₁   V₄

II   VL   V₂   V₅

III   VF   V₃   V₆

Note: Normal axis
S wave exceeds R wave in V₁
Inverted T waves in V₁–V₂.

There is obviously some variation in the age at which the apparent right ventricular hypertrophy disappears, but all its features other than the inverted T waves in V_1 and V_2 should have disappeared by the age of 2 years. The T wave 'abnormalities' may persist until the age of 10 years.

NORMAL ECG: AGE 5 YEARS

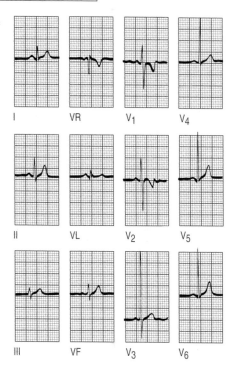

Note: Normal axis
Normal QRS complexes in the V leads
T waves inverted in V_1–V_2.

By the age of 10 years, the ECG should have taken on the adult pattern.

NORMAL ECG: AGE 10 YEARS

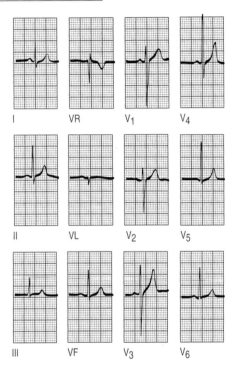

Note: The record is indistinguishable from that of a normal adult.

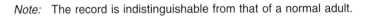

In general, if the infant ECG pattern persists beyond the age of 2 years, then right ventricular hypertrophy is indeed present. If the normal adult pattern is present in the first year of life, then left ventricular hypertrophy is present.

SPECIFIC ECG ABNORMALITIES IN HEALTHY PEOPLE

The ECG findings we have discussed so far can all be considered to be within the normal range. Certain findings are undoubtedly abnormal as far as the ECG is concerned, yet do occur in apparently healthy people.

The frequency with which various abnormalities are detected depends on the population studied: most abnormalities are found least often in healthy young people recruited to the armed services, and become progressively more common in populations of increasing age. An exception to this rule is that frequent ventricular extrasystoles are very common in pregnancy. The frequency of right and left bundle branch block has been found to be 0.3% and 0.1% respectively in populations of young service recruits, but in older working populations these abnormalities have been detected in 2% and 0.7% respectively of apparently healthy people.

Table 1.1 shows the frequency with which the more common ECG abnormalities were encountered in a large survey of civil servants. All the abnormalities, except the Wolff-Parkinson-White

Table 1.1 Prevalence of the more common ECG abnormalities in 18 000 civil servants (rates per 1000) (after Rose et al 1978 British Heart Journal 40: 636–643)

	Age		
	40–49	50–59	60–64
Frequent ventricular extrasystoles	8	14	26
Atrial fibrillation	2	4	11
Left axis deviation	23	32	49
First degree block	18	26	33
Left bundle branch block	9	16	31
Abnormal T wave inversion	9	54	76
WPW syndrome	0.3	0.2	0

(WPW) syndrome, which is congenital (Ch. 2), were found more frequently with increasing age. This suggests that the various abnormalities are all indicators of heart disease. The survey was of a working population, but some individuals had symptoms of heart disease and of course these were more common in the older age group. This sort of survey shows how difficult it is to define the precise range of 'normality' in the ECG.

WHAT TO DO

When an apparently healthy subject has an ECG record that appears abnormal, the most important thing is not to cause unnecessary alarm. There are four questions to ask:

1. Does the ECG really come from that individual? If so, is he or she really asymptomatic and are the findings of the physical examination really normal?
2. Is the ECG really abnormal or is it within the normal range?
3. If the ECG is indeed abnormal, what are the implications for the patient?
4. What further investigations are needed?

The range of normality

Normal variations in the P waves, QRS complexes and T waves have been described in detail. T wave changes usually give the most trouble in terms of ECG interpretation, because changes in repolarization occur in many different circumstances, and in any individual variations in T wave morphology can occur from day to day. Below are listed some of the ECG patterns that can be accepted as normal in healthy patients, and some that must be regarded with suspicion.

Always normal:
- Sinus arrhythmia
- Supraventricular extrasystoles
- Incomplete right bundle branch block
- 'High take-off' ST segment
- T wave inversion in lead III but not VF
- T wave inversion in VR and V_1.

Not necessarily indicative of heart disease:
- Ventricular extrasystoles
- Left or right axis deviation
- Right bundle branch block
- T wave inversion in leads other than III, VR, V_1
- Non-specific ST segment changes.

The prognosis of patients with an abnormal ECG

In general, the prognosis is related to the patient's clinical history and to the findings on physical examination, rather than to the ECG. An abnormal ECG is much more significant in a patient with symptoms and signs of heart disease than it is in a truly healthy subject.

In the absence of any other evidence of heart disease, the prognosis of an individual with one of the more common ECG abnormalities is as follows.

Conduction defects

Of the conduction defects, first degree block (especially when the PR interval is only slightly prolonged) has little effect on prognosis. Second and third degree block indicate heart disease and the prognosis is worse, though the congenital form of complete block is less serious than the acquired form in adults. Left anterior hemiblock has a good prognosis, as does right bundle branch block. The presence of left bundle branch block in the absence of other manifestations of cardiac disease is associated with about a 30% increase in the risk of death, compared with that of individuals with a normal ECG. The risk of death doubles if a subject known to have a normal ECG develops left bundle branch block (LBBB), even if there are no symptoms. Bifascicular block seldom progresses to complete block, but is always an indication of underlying heart disease and the prognosis is therefore relatively poor.

Arrhythmias

Among the arrhythmias, supraventricular extrasystoles are of no importance whatsoever. Ventricular extrasystoles are almost universal but when frequent or multiform they indicate populations with an increased risk of death, presumably because in a proportion of people they indicate sub-clinical heart disease. The increased risk to an individual is, however, minimal and there is no evidence that treating ventricular extrasystoles prolongs survival. Atrial fibrillation is frequently the result of rheumatic or ischaemic heart disease or cardiomyopathy, and the prognosis is then relatively poor. In about one-third of individuals with atrial fibrillation no cardiac disease can be demonstrated, but in such people the risk of death is increased three- or four-fold, and the risk of stroke perhaps 10 fold, compared with people of the same age who are in sinus rhythm.

Further investigations

Complex and expensive investigations are seldom justified in asymptomatic patients whose hearts are clinically normal but who have been found to have an abnormal ECG.

A chest X-ray should probably be taken in patients with bundle branch block or atrial fibrillation, to provide an accurate estimate of heart size. Since left bundle branch block may indicate a dilated cardiomyopathy, an echocardiogram can be recorded to assess left ventricular function. Echocardiography may be diagnostically useful but therapeutically unhelpful if anterior T wave inversion raises the possibility of hypertrophic cardiomyopathy.

Patients with frequent ventricular extrasystoles may merit a chest X-ray and the measurement of their haemoglobin level, but nothing else.

In patients with atrial fibrillation an echocardiogram is useful for defining, or excluding, structural abnormalities, and for studying left ventricular function. An echocardiogram is indicated if there is anything that might suggest rheumatic heart disease. Since atrial fibrillation can be the only manifestation of thyrotoxicosis, thyroid function must be checked. Atrial fibrillation may be the result of alcoholism and this may be denied by the patient, so it may be fair to check liver function also.

Treatment of asymptomatic ECG abnormalities

It is always the patient who should be treated, not the ECG. The prognosis of patients with complete heart block is improved by permanent pacing, but that of patients with other degrees of block is not. Ventricular extrasystoles should not be treated because of the risk of pro-arrhythmic effects of anti-arrhythmic drugs. Atrial fibrillation need not be treated if the ventricular rate is reasonable, but anticoagulation must be considered in all cases. In the case of patients with valve disease and atrial fibrillation, however, anticoagulant treatment is essential.

A full ECG is shown on the next two pages as an aid to pattern recognition. Below it is the appropriate description and interpretation.

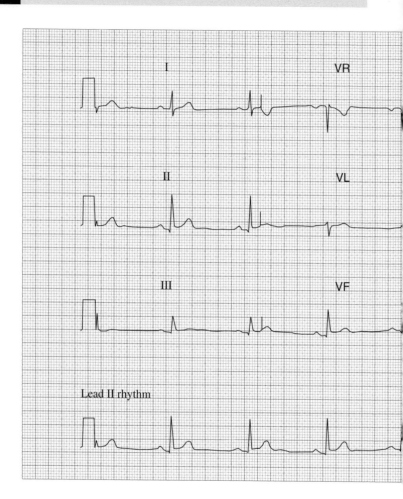

This ECG was recorded from a 45-year-old man at a routine medical examination.

The ECG shows:
- Sinus rhythm, with normal conduction intervals
- Normal axis

- QRS complexes of normal width, height and depth
- Normal ST segments and T waves.

Interpretation:

Normal record.

CHAPTER 2

The ECG in patients with palpitations and syncope

The ECG is of paramount importance for the diagnosis of arrhythmias: no other investigation can substitute for it. Many arrhythmias are not noticed by the patient and they are common in patients who are monitored in a Coronary Care Unit (CCU) following an acute myocardial infarction. However, arrhythmias do sometimes cause symptoms – although in many cases these are transient, and the patient is completely well at the time he or she consults a doctor. Under such circumstances, obtaining an ECG during a symptomatic episode is the only certain way of making a diagnosis, but as always the history and physical examination are also extremely important.

THE CLINICAL HISTORY

A cardiac arrhythmia can cause several different symptoms. The patient may become aware of an abnormal heartbeat – the symptom of 'palpitations'. The arrhythmia may interfere with cardiac function and cause dizziness or collapse (syncope), due to hypotension and poor cerebral blood flow. It can also cause breathlessness, due to heart failure. Poor coronary blood flow may cause angina.

The main purpose of the history and physical examination is to help in deciding whether a patient's symptoms could be the result of an arrhythmia, and whether the patient has a cardiac or other disease that might cause an arrhythmia.

Sinus rhythm

People are not normally aware of their heartbeat but everyone notices the rapid, regular, and forceful beat of sinus tachycardia due to exercise, excitement, or fright. Usually the relationship of such 'palpitations' to a precipitating cause will be obvious, and the individual will not feel the need to seek medical advice. However, anxious individuals may go to their doctor complaining of palpitations and a carefully-taken history will reveal an enhanced awareness of, and alarm about, a normal heartbeat. As well as the circumstances in which such 'attacks' occur, the patient will describe a progressive acceleration of heart rate rather than a sudden onset of palpitations. Anxiety-induced sinus tachycardia does not usually compromise cardiac function, though patients with ischaemic heart disease may develop angina. A patient with anxiety-induced sinus tachycardia may complain of breathlessness and dizziness due to hyperventilation, but this can be identified from the typical tingling sensation that this causes around the mouth and in the fingers.

Sinus tachycardia is the appropriate response of the circulatory system to anaemia, loss of circulating volume, and thyrotoxicosis, and these possible diagnoses must be kept in mind while the history is being taken and the patient examined.

Extrasystoles

Palpitations due to extrasystoles are very common. The patient's description usually makes the diagnosis easy: the heart 'skips a beat', 'jumps into the throat' or 'seems to stop'. Extrasystoles are usually single, but may be repeated frequently, and patients tend to notice them particularly when lying in bed at night. Extrasystoles do not cause the symptoms associated with poor cardiac function. Physical examination may reveal an irregularity of the heartbeat, and the only rhythm likely to be confused with extrasystoles is atrial fibrillation. It is not possible to distinguish between supraventricular and ventricular extrasystoles, either from the history or from the examination.

Paroxysmal tachycardia

An episode of paroxysmal tachycardia typically causes the sudden onset of palpitations. The patient will usually be able to recognize whether the heartbeat is regular or not, and with instruction may be able to count the heart rate. This is valuable information, for a rate of less than 140 per minute is usually due to sinus tachycardia. Any unprovoked episode of palpitations associated with chest pain, breathlessness or dizziness must be considered to be due to an arrhythmia until proved otherwise. If the attack ends abruptly it is almost certainly due to an arrhythmia, though frequently patients will describe episodes of paroxysmal tachycardia as 'dying away'. Table 2.1 shows how the diagnosis of sinus tachycardia or paroxysmal tachycardia may be made from the patient's symptoms.

Table 2.1 Diagnosis of sinus tachycardia or paroxysmal tachycardia from the patient's symptoms

Symptoms	Sinus tachycardia	Paroxysmal tachycardia
Timing of initial attack	Attacks probably began recently	Attacks probably began in teens or early adult life
Associations of attack	Exercise, anxiety	Usually no associations, but occasionally exercise-induced
Rate of start of palpitations	Slow build-up	Sudden onset
Rate of end of palpitations	'Die away'	Classically sudden, but often 'die away'
Heart rate	< 140 per minute	> 160 per minute
Associated symptoms	Paraesthesia due to hyperventilation	Chest pain, breathlessness, dizziness, syncope
Ways of terminating attacks	Relaxation	Breath holding, Valsalva's manoeuvre

Dizziness and syncope

The most common cause of syncope is simple fainting. This is best recognized from the situations in which attacks occur; the patient is always standing at the time, often in a hot and crowded room or in a situation of emotional stress. A description of the attack from a witness is always helpful: in a faint, the patient is pale and the pulse may be difficult to find, but if accurately described the heart rate is slow, the rhythm being sinus bradycardia due to vagal overactivity. Recovery occurs within seconds of lying flat.

Syncope can also result from postural hypotension and this is particularly important in old people, in patients taking hypotensive drugs and in those with abnormalities of the autonomic control of the circulation due to diabetes, Parkinsonism, or idiopathic degeneration of the autonomic nervous system (the Shy-Drager syndrome).

Attacks of dizziness or syncope can occur in patients with cardiovascular disease without any abnormality of cardiac rhythm if there is physical obstruction to blood flow. Important causes of such symptoms are aortic stenosis and hypertrophic cardiomyopathy (when dizziness is usually associated with physical activity), intracardiac tumours such as an atrial myxoma, and pulmonary embolism. In a young woman, exercise-induced syncope may be caused by severe pulmonary hypertension, sometimes the result of repeated small pulmonary emboli that themselves have caused few symptoms.

The main difficulty in reaching a diagnosis, however, is to differentiate syncopal attacks due to arrhythmias from various sorts of epilepsy due to neurological disease, because any syncopal attack due to cerebral hypoxia can cause a grand mal fit. The classic syncopal attack due to an arrhythmia is the 'Stokes-Adams' attack associated with complete heart block: here a critical reduction in ventricular rate reduces cardiac output and cerebral flow to a point at which sudden loss of consciousness occurs. The patient appears very pale, but flushes red on recovery. Between attacks the patient may be well, but may describe symptoms of heart failure due to a slow rate. Epileptic attacks due to neurological disease are easy to recognize if there are any features indicating that a particular region of the brain is involved, or if there are any associated neurological symptoms between attacks. Frequently, however, this is not the case and differentiation between cardiovascular and neurological disease depends on evidence from examination or from evidence of disease in one or other system.

PHYSICAL EXAMINATION

The aim of the physical examination is to find out whether the patient has an arrhythmia and whether there are any signs of cardiovascular disease that might cause an arrhythmia. An anxious patient complaining of palpitations due to sinus tachycardia will often have a relatively high heart rate (up to 130 per minute), the skin will be cold and sweaty and the systolic blood pressure will be high. The main differential diagnosis is thyrotoxicosis, which will usually be associated with a goitre and the characteristic warm skin, lid lag, and proptosis. Intermittent attacks of sinus tachycardia occur with phaeochromocytomata, and this diagnosis must be considered when the blood pressure is elevated.

Usually patients with a paroxysmal arrhythmia will be seen when in sinus rhythm, although by chance an arrhythmia may be present at the time of examination. The presence of an abnormality of heart rate or rhythm may give a clue to the nature of paroxysmal attacks. For example, patients with Stokes-Adams attacks may be found to be in complete heart block, which can be recognized clinically from the slow and regular heart rate and from the presence of 'cannon' waves in the jugular venous pulse. In young people, a slow heart rate may be due to sinoatrial disease (the 'sick sinus syndrome'), and this can be associated with a paroxysmal tachycardia.

When the heart is in sinus rhythm with a normal rate, it is necessary to look for some signs of cardiac or (in the case of syncopal attacks) neurological disease. In particular, the blood pressure should be measured when the patient is lying down and also when standing, the position of the apex beat should be identified, and the presence of right or left ventricular hypertrophy noted. On auscultation it is the presence of aortic and mitral stenosis that is most likely to indicate the cause of syncope or palpitations. Evidence of heart disease of any type makes an arrhythmia a possible cause of palpitations and syncope, but of course arrhythmias commonly cause problems in people whose hearts appear normal between attacks.

Table 2.2 lists some of the clinical problems that can be associated with tachycardias, and so cause the patient to complain of palpitations. Remember that very fast heart rates – especially with ventricular tachycardia – can cause dizziness and syncope, and the patient may sometimes be unaware of the abnormal rhythm.

Table 2.2 Conditions associated with palpitations

Cardiac rhythm	Underlying cause
Extrasystoles	Normal heart Any cardiac disease Anaemia
Sinus tachycardia	Normal heart Anxiety Anaemia Acute blood loss Pregnancy Lung disease CO_2 retention Pulmonary embolus Phaeochromocytoma
Atrial fibrillation	Rheumatic heart disease Thyrotoxicosis Ischaemic heart disease Cardiomyopathy Alcoholism Apparently normal heart with 'lone atrial fibrillation'
Supraventricular tachycardia	Pre-excitation syndromes Apparently normal heart
Ventricular tachycardia	Acute myocardial infarction Ischaemic heart disease Cardiomyopathy (hypertrophic or dilated) Long QT syndrome Myocarditis Drugs Apparently normal heart – idiopathic

Table 2.3 lists some of the clinical causes of syncope, and the cardiac rhythms with which attacks might be associated.

Table 2.3 Conditions associated with syncope

Cardiac rhythm	Underlying cause
Sinus rhythm	Neurological diseases, including epilepsy Vagal overactivity — simple faint — acute myocardial infarction Postural hypotension — blood loss — hypotensive drugs — Addison's disease — autonomic dysfunction Circulatory obstruction — aortic or pulmonary stenosis — hypertrophic cardiomyopathy — pulmonary embolus — pulmonary hypertension — atrial myxoma Drugs — beta-blockers
Atrial fibrillation with slow ventricular rate	Rheumatic heart disease Ischaemic heart disease Cardiomyopathies Drugs — digoxin — beta-blockers — verapamil — amiodarone
Sick sinus syndrome	Congenital Familial Idiopathic Ischaemic heart disease Rheumatic heart disease Cardiomyopathy Amyloidosis Collagen diseases

Table 2.3 (*cont'd*)

Cardiac rhythm	Underlying cause
	Myocarditis
	Drugs
	– lithium
Second or third degree block	Idiopathic (fibrosis)
	Congenital
	Ischaemia
	Aortic valve calcification
	Surgery or trauma
	Tumours in the His bundle
	Drugs
	– digoxin
	– beta-blockers

THE ECG IN PATIENTS WITH PALPITATIONS AND SYNCOPE

It is only possible to make a confident diagnosis that an arrhythmia is the cause of palpitations or syncope if an EGC recording of the arrhythmia can be obtained, and if it can be shown that the occurrence of the arrhythmia coincides with the patient's symptoms. If the patient is asymptomatic at the time of examination, it may be worth arranging for an ECG to be recorded immediately during an attack of palpitations, or it may be worth recording the ECG continuously for 24 hours on a tape recorder (the 'Holter' technique) in the hope that an episode of the arrhythmia will be detected. This is relatively time-consuming for technicians and is therefore expensive – it is only worthwhile if there are reasonable clinical grounds for suspecting an arrhythmia and if the episodes occur sufficiently frequently for there to be a reasonable chance of an arrhythmia being recorded.

THE ECG WHEN THE PATIENT IS ASYMPTOMATIC

Patients who complain of palpitations or syncope are often completely well when they see a doctor, but even then the resting ECG can be very helpful.

Syncope due to cardiac causes other than arrhythmias

Although the main use of the ECG is to diagnose arrhythmias, occasionally ECG abnormalities will be seen indicating that syncopal attacks may be due to cardiovascular disease other than an arrhythmia.

The presence of marked left ventricular hypertrophy will suggest the possibility that syncope is due to aortic stenosis.

LV HYPERTROPHY DUE TO AORTIC STENOSIS

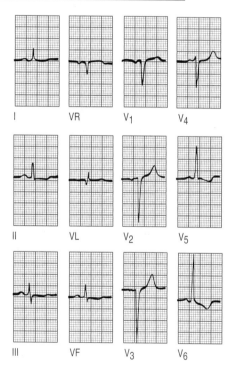

Note: Tall R wave in V_6, deep S waves in V_2–V_3
Inverted T waves in leads II and V_5–V_6.

ECG evidence of severe right ventricular hypertrophy will raise the possibility of thromboembolic pulmonary hypertension.

RV HYPERTROPHY DUE TO MULTIPLE PULMONARY EMBOLI

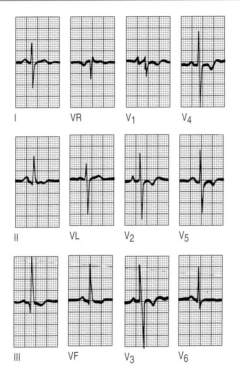

Note: Sinus rhythm
Peaked P waves
Right axis deviation
Inverted T waves in V_1–V_5
S wave in V_6
The only 'missing' feature of right ventricular hypertrophy is a dominant R wave in V_1 (see Ch. 4).

However, the ECG may suggest that an arrhythmia is likely even when the patient is asymptomatic and physical examination is normal.

Patients with possible tachycardia

Mitral stenosis

Mitral stenosis is an important cause of atrial fibrillation, but it is possible to miss hearing the characteristic diastolic murmur. ECG evidence of left atrial hypertrophy may indicate that atrial fibrillation is the cause of intermittent irregular and fast palpitations.

MITRAL STENOSIS

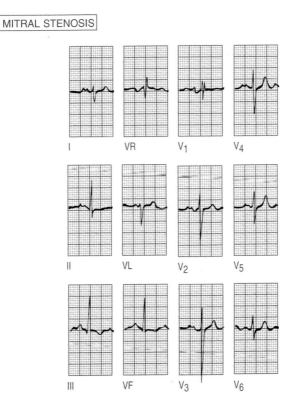

I   VR   V₁   V₄

II   VL   V₂   V₅

III   VF   V₃   V₆

Note: Sinus rhythm
Broad and notched P waves suggest left atrial hypertrophy
Right axis deviation and S wave in V₆ suggest right
ventricular hypertrophy
The partial RBBB is not significant.

Pre-excitation syndromes

In the pre-excitation syndromes there are abnormal pathways connecting the atria and ventricles, which form an anatomical basis for re-entry tachycardia (see Ch. 6).

In the Wolff-Parkinson-White syndrome, an accessory pathway can be identified microscopically: this is usually between the left atrium and left ventricle, but sometimes there is an abnormal connection between the right atrium and ventricle. In either case, the normal atrioventricular nodal delay is bypassed, so the PR interval is short and ventricular activation is initially abnormal. However, excitation spreading through the AV node and bundle of His causes normal (late) ventricular excitation. A short PR interval is thus followed by a slurred upstroke of the R wave, and this slurred wave is called a 'delta wave'.

In the case of a left-side accessory pathway, the ECG shows a dominant R wave in V_1, and superficially resembles right ventricular hypertrophy. This is called a 'Type A' pattern.

WOLFF-PARKINSON-WHITE SYNDROME

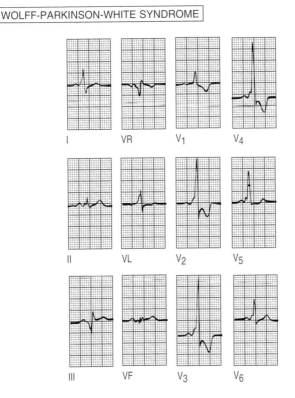

Note: Short PR interval
Slurred upstroke of R wave (delta wave), seen in all leads but especially in V_2–V_6
Dominant R wave in V_1
Inverted T waves in V_1–V_4.

When the accessory pathway is on the right side of the heart there is no dominant R wave in V_1, and this pattern is called 'Type B'.

WOLFF-PARKINSON-WHITE SYNDROME

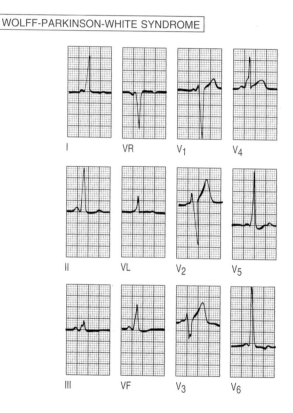

Note: Short PR interval
The delta wave is most obvious in V_4.

Where there is a bypass causing rapid conduction from the atria to the bundle of His itself, there is also a short PR interval but the QRS complex is entirely normal; this is the Lown-Ganong-Levine syndrome.

LOWN-GANONG-LEVINE SYNDROME

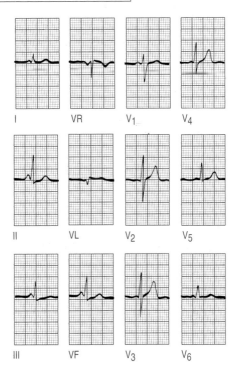

Note: Short PR interval
Narrow and normal QRS complexes.

Pre-excitation syndromes are found in approximately one in every 3000 healthy young people, but only half of them ever have an episode of tachycardia, and many of these only have very occasional attacks. During an episode of re-entry tachycardia, the QRS complex is usually narrow and the pattern resembles a junctional tachycardia; the presence of a pre-excitation syndrome may not be suspected.

Broad complex tachycardias also occur in patients with the WPW syndrome. Although the ECG may resemble ventricular tachycardia, in most cases the underlying rhythm is probably atrial fibrillation with anomalous atrioventricular conduction. This is a serious arrhythmia, because ventricular fibrillation may occur. The physiological mechanisms involved in the tachycardias of the WPW syndrome are discussed in Chapter 6.

TACHYCARDIAS IN WPW SYNDROME

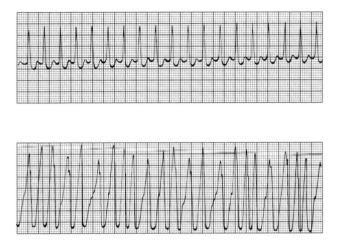

Note: Upper and lower traces show a narrow complex and a
wide complex tachycardia respectively. In the lower trace,
the marked irregularity and variation in the complexes
suggest that the rhythm is atrial fibrillation. The underlying
diagnosis of WPW syndrome is not apparent in either
case.

The long QT syndrome

Delayed repolarization occurs for a variety of reasons, and occasionally for no apparent reason. Causes of a prolonged QT interval and torsades de pointes ventricular tachycardia include:

- Congenital
  - Jervell-Lange-Nielson syndrome
  - Romano-Ward syndrome
- Anti-arrhythmic drugs
  - quinidine
  - procainamide
  - disopyramide
  - amiodarone
  - sotalol
- Other drugs
  - ketanserin
  - tricyclic antidepressants
  - erythromycin
  - thioridazine
- Plasma electrolyte abnormality
  - low potassium
  - low magnesium
  - low calcium.

In the long QT syndrome, the ECG shows a prolonged QT interval, but this in itself does not impair cardiac function or cause symptoms.

LONG QT SYNDROME

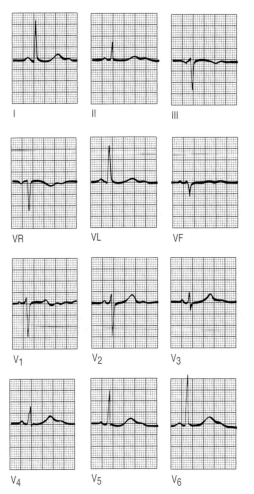

I   II   III

VR   VL   VF

V_1 V_2 V_3

V_4 V_5 V_6

Note: Sinus rhythm, with a normal PR interval and a normal
cardiac axis
The T wave is followed by a U wave
(The QT interval is 600 ms.)

The prolonged QT interval is, however, sometimes associated with paroxysmal ventricular tachycardia and characteristically this involves a continuous change from upright to downward complexes. This is called 'torsades de pointes'.

The congenital long QT syndromes cause episodes of loss of consciousness in children, often at times of increased sympathetic nervous system activity. Such episodes occur in about 8% of affected subjects each year, and the annual rate of death due to arrhythmias is about 1% of patients with a long QT syndrome.

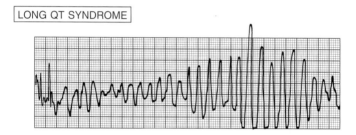

LONG QT SYNDROME

Note: This ECG is from the same patient as the record on page 69. The patient had frequent episodes of ventricular tachycardia of the torsades de pointes type.

Patients with possible bradycardias

When the patient is asymptomatic, an intermittent bradycardia can be suspected if the ECG shows any evidence of a conduction defect. Nevertheless, it must be remembered that conduction defects are quite common in healthy people, and their presence may be coincidental (see Ch. 1).

However, when a patient complains of syncopal attacks, ECG changes that would be ignored in a healthy person take on a greater significance. First and second degree block may point to intermittent complete block.

1st DEGREE BLOCK

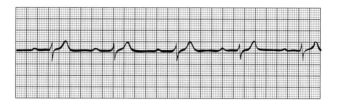

Note: Sinus rhythm
PR interval is constant at 320 ms.

2nd DEGREE BLOCK (MOBITZ TYPE 2)

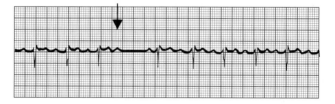

Note: Sinus rhythm, with a normal PR interval
One P wave (arrowed) is not followed by a QRS complex.

2nd DEGREE BLOCK (2:1)

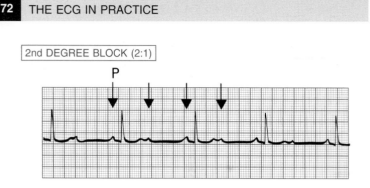

Note: The conducted beats have a normal PR interval, but
alternate P waves are not followed by a QRS complex.

   The combination of bundle branch block and first degree block
suggests that conduction may also fail intermittently in the
remaining bundle branch.

1st DEGREE BLOCK AND BUNDLE BRANCH BLOCK

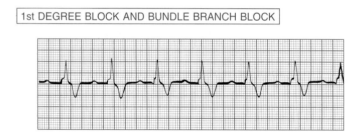

Note: PR interval 280 ms, indicating first degree block
Broad QRS complexes and inverted T waves indicate
bundle branch block, but it is not possible to tell from a
single lead which branch is affected.

Intermittent complete heart block may also be suspected when there is evidence of abnormal conduction in two of the three main divisions of the bundle of His (the right bundle and the anterior or posterior divisions of the left bundle branch). Such 'bifascicular block' is indicated by the combination of right bundle branch block and marked left axis deviation.

BIFASCICULAR BLOCK

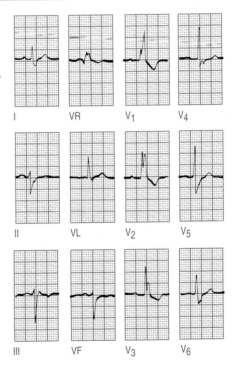

Note: Sinus rhythm
Left axis deviation
QRS complex shows RSR^1 pattern in V_1, indicating right bundle branch block (RBBB).

So even when the patient is asymptomatic the ECG can be very helpful: Table 2.4 lists some of the things to look for and to think about.

Table 2.4 ECG features between attacks of palpitations or syncope

ECG appearance	Possible cause of symptoms
ECG completely normal	Symptoms may not be due to a primary arrhythmia – consider anxiety, epilepsy, atrial myxoma or carotid sinus hypersensitivity
ECGs that suggest cardiac disease	Left ventricular hypertrophy: aortic stenosis Right ventricular hypertrophy: pulmonary hypertension Anterior T wave inversion: hypertrophic cardiomyopathy
ECGs that suggest intermittent tachy-arrhythmia	Left atrial hypertrophy: mitral stenosis, so possibly atrial fibrillation Pre-excitation syndromes Long QT syndrome Flat T wave suggests hypokalaemia Digitalis effect: ?digitalis toxicity
ECGs that suggest intermittent brady-arrhythmia	Second degree block First degree block plus bundle branch block Digitalis effect

THE ECG WHEN THE PATIENT HAS SYMPTOMS

Several arrhythmias are of considerable physiological interest but do not cause symptoms: these will be discussed in Chapter 6. If an ECG can be recorded at the time when the patient has palpitations, dizziness or syncope then there can be little doubt about the relationship between the symptoms and the cardiac rhythm.

Sinus rhythm in patients with symptoms

When sinus tachycardia results from anxiety, heart rates of up to 150 per minute are not uncommon. The rhythm may be mistaken for an atrial tachycardia, but pressure on the carotid sinus will cause transient slowing of the heart rate and the P waves will became more obvious.

Marked sinus bradycardia is characteristic of athletic training, but it is also part of the cause of symptoms in fainting (the 'vasovagal' attack), and it may also contribute to hypotension and heart failure in patients with an inferior myocardial infarction.

Extrasystoles in patients with symptoms

An ECG is necessary to differentiate between supraventricular and ventricular extrasystoles.

When extrasystoles have a supraventricular origin, the QRS complex is narrow and both it and the T wave have the same configuration as in the sinus beat. Atrial extrasystoles have abnormal P waves; junctional extrasystoles either have a P wave very close to the QRS complex (in front of it or behind it) or have no visible P waves.

ATRIAL EXTRASYSTOLE

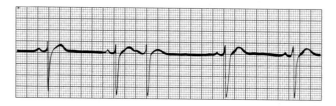

JUNCTIONAL (AV NODAL) EXTRASYSTOLE

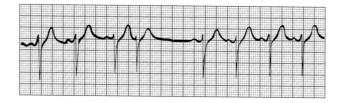

Note: An atrial extrasystole has an abnormally-shaped P wave
A junctional (AV nodal) extrasystole usually shows no P wave.

Ventricular extrasystoles produce wide QRS complexes of abnormal shape, and the T wave is also usually abnormal. No P waves are present.

VENTRICULAR EXTRASYSTOLES

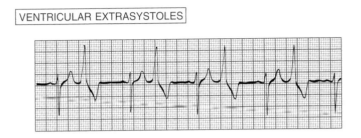

Note: Each sinus beat is followed by a beat with no P wave, a wide QRS complex and an inverted T wave. This is sometimes called 'bigeminy'.

The corresponding 'escape beats' have the same characteristics, but occur late rather than early (see Ch. 6).

When a ventricular extrasystole appears on the upstroke of the T wave of the preceding beat, the 'R on T' phenomenon is said to be present. This can initiate ventricular fibrillation, but usually it does not do so.

R ON T PHENOMENON

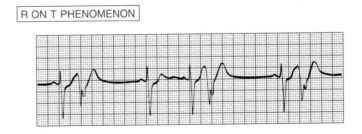

Note: Ventricular extrasystoles occur near the peak of the preceding T wave.

TACHYCARDIAS IN PATIENTS WITH SYMPTOMS

The pathophysiology of tachycardias is discussed in Chapter 6. Here we can be concerned with their diagnosis and management.

Narrow complex tachycardias

A tachycardia can be described as 'narrow complex' if the QRS complex duration is less than 120 ms.

Properly speaking, sinus, atrial and junctional arrhythmias are all supraventricular, but the term 'supraventricular tachycardia' is often inappropriately used interchangeably with 'junctional tachycardia'. All these supraventricular rhythms have QRS complexes of normal shape and width, and the T waves have the same shape as in the sinus beat.

Atrial tachycardia

In atrial tachycardia, P waves are present, but they have an abnormal shape. They are sometimes hidden in the T wave of the preceding beat.

ATRIAL TACHYCARDIA

Note: Two sinus beats are followed by a sudden change of heart rate. In the tachycardia, P waves can be seen as humps on the T waves of the preceding beats.

In atrial tachycardia, the P wave rate is in the range 130–250 per minute. When the atrial rate exceeds about 180 per minute, physiological block will occur in the atrioventricular node, so that the ventricular rate becomes half that of the atria. The main significance of atrial tachycardia with 2:1 block is that it is characteristic of digitalis toxicity.

Atrial flutter

In atrial flutter, the atrial rate is about 300 per minute and the P waves form a continuous 'sawtoothed' line. As the AV node usually fails to conduct all the P waves, the relationship between P waves and QRS complexes is usually 2:1, 3:1 or 4:1.

ATRIAL FLUTTER

2:1 block

4:1 block

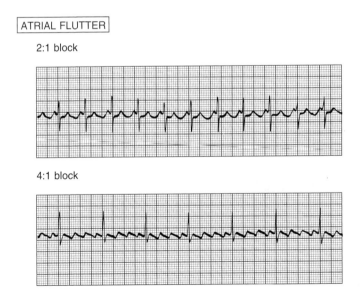

Note: In atrial flutter with 2:1 block, a P wave may be confused with a T wave. With 4:1 block, the flutter waves are obvious.

With 2:1 block, the 'sawtooth' may not be obvious in all leads and as always it is best to examine a 12-lead cardiogram and diagnose the rhythm from the lead in which the P waves are most obvious.

ATRIAL FLUTTER

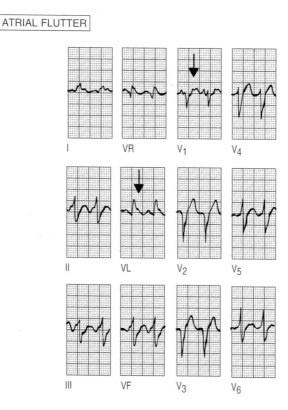

Note: In this record the P waves are most obvious in leads VL and V_1.

If the ventricular rate is rapid, carotid sinus pressure will usually increase the block at the AV node and make the 'sawtooth' more obvious (see p. 266).

Junctional or atrioventricular re-entry tachycardia

Junctional tachycardia is caused by re-entry of the electrical impulse via a double conducting channel within, or very close to, the AV node (see p. 264). 'Junctional' tachycardia is therefore now usually called 'atrioventricular re-entry' (AVRE) tachycardia. In this rhythm, no P waves can be seen. Carotid sinus pressure either reverts the heart to sinus rhythm or has no effect.

AVRE (JUNCTIONAL) TACHYCARDIA

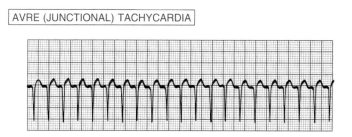

Note: Regular, narrow QRS complexes at 180 per minute
No P waves visible.

Atrial fibrillation

In atrial fibrillation, disorganized atrial activity causes the P waves
to disappear, and the ECG baseline becomes totally irregular. At
times, atrial activity may become sufficiently synchronized for a
'flutter-like' pattern to appear, but this rapidly breaks up. The QRS
complexes are totally irregular.

ATRIAL FIBRILLATION

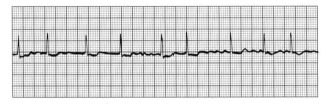

Note: Variable atrial activity with 'flutter-like' waves at times
Irregular narrow QRS complexes.

The QRS complex may become regular, and this is seen with
digitalis toxicity. It is important to remember that totally regular and
slow QRS complexes may indicate complete heart block, and that
this can occur in the presence of atrial fibrillation.

ATRIAL FIBRILLATION WITH COMPLETE BLOCK

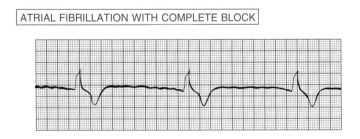

Note: Variable atrial activity
Regular, wide QRS complexes at 30 per minute.

Broad complex rhythms

Slow broad complex rhythms include complete block with a ventricular focus controlling ventricular activity, and sinus bradycardia, atrial fibrillation or some other supraventricular rhythm with bundle branch block.

A tachycardia can be described as 'broad complex' if the QRS complex duration exceeds 120 ms. In the context of acute myocardial infarction, broad complex tachycardias are usually ventricular in origin, but in other circumstances they can be either ventricular, or supraventricular with bundle branch block.

Rhythms of ventricular origin with a rate of less than 120 per minute are best described as 'accelerated idioventricular rhythm', and the term 'ventricular tachycardia' is used only when the rate exceeds 120 per minute.

VENTRICULAR TACHYCARDIA

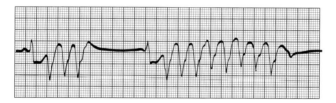

Note: A sinus beat is followed by three ventricular beats, at 210 per minute

A second sinus beat is followed by a run of ventricular tachycardia.

A supraventricular tachycardia can be associated with broad QRS complexes either because of bundle branch block or because of the Wolff-Parkinson-White syndrome.

Differentiation between broad complex tachycardias

Differentiation between broad complex tachycardias of supraventricular and ventricular origin can be difficult, and it is essential to remember that the patient's clinical state is completely unhelpful: rhythms of either type may be well tolerated for long periods, but either can cause a haemodynamic disturbance with angina, heart failure or dizziness due to hypotension. The patient's state depends on the heart rate and the degree of underlying cardiac disease, not on the origin of the arrhythmia.

A supraventricular origin for a broad complex tachycardia can only safely be diagnosed when there is intermittent sinus rhythm which produces the same QRS complex configuration as does the tachycardia.

SINUS RHYTHM WITH BIFASCICULAR BLOCK

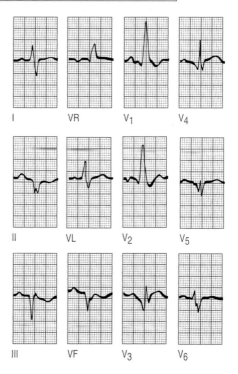

I   VR V_1 V_4

II   VL V_2 V_5

III   VF V_3 V_6

Note: Sinus rhythm with left axis deviation
Broad QRS complexes with an RSR[1] pattern in V_1 and a
deep notched S wave in V_6 indicate RBBB.

SUPRAVENTRICULAR TACHYCARDIA

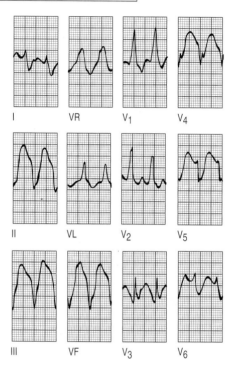

Note: Traces from the same patient as those shown on the preceding page, but during an episode of tachycardia. Unless it were known that the same ECG appearance was present in sinus rhythm, it might have been assumed that this is ventricular tachycardia. Although superficially these traces look different from those on p. 85, in fact the cardiac axis is the same and a comparison of the QRS complexes in each lead in the two sets of traces shows their similarity.

If the appearance of the ECG during the tachycardia is quite different from that during sinus rhythm, the origin of the tachycardia may be ventricular, or may be supraventricular with bundle branch block: bundle branch block can be rate-dependent, and so may only appear in response to a supraventricular tachycardia.

| JUNCTIONAL TACHYCARDIA WITH BUNDLE BRANCH BLOCK |

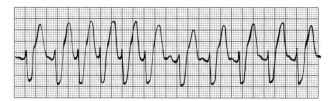

Note: This record shows a single sinus beat with a broad QRS complex, followed by five beats without P waves but with the same broad QRS complex. Sinus rhythm is then restored. This arrhythmia is junctional tachycardia with bundle branch block.

There are, however, some features of the ECG that can be used to distinguish supraventricular from ventricular rhythms. Unfortunately some of these differentiating features are seldom seen, and those that are seen are not infallible. It is, therefore, important whenever possible to have a full 12-lead record taken during the tachycardia, and to look for the following features:

1. The presence of P waves
2. The QRS complex duration
3. QRS complex regularity
4. The cardiac axis
5. QRS complex configuration
6. The presence of fusion and capture beats.

Presence of P waves

A 12-lead ECG during the tachycardia is important because P waves may be visible in some leads but not in others.

Occasionally it may be possible to identify P waves with a slower rate than the QRS complexes.

VENTRICULAR TACHYCARDIA

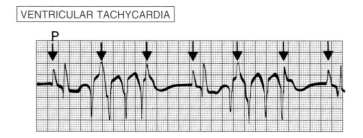

Note: A single sinus beat is followed by a broad complex tachycardia. During the tachycardia P waves can still be seen at a normal rate, so the broad complex tachycardia must have a ventricular origin.

QRS complex duration

A broad complex tachycardia is likely to have a ventricular origin if the QRS complex duration exceeds 160 ms, because bundle branch block complexes are usually of 120–160 ms duration. However, pre-excitation may cause very wide QRS complexes. Conversely, a ventricular tachycardia originating in the conducting tissue can have a complex with a duration of less than 120 ms.

QRS complex regularity

Ventricular tachycardia is usually regular, but so is a junctional tachycardia with bundle branch block. A very irregular wide complex tachycardia is usually due to atrial fibrillation plus a conduction defect, or to atrial flutter with variable block plus a conduction defect. Pre-excitation with atrial fibrillation can produce a similar pattern. However, polymorphic ventricular tachycardia and torsades de pointes ventricular tachycardia are both irregular.

Cardiac axis

Left axis deviation, especially when associated with right bundle branch block, usually indicates a tachycardia of ventricular origin. Any axis change compared with that of sinus rhythm also suggests that the tachycardia is ventricular in origin.

QRS complex configuration

The QRS complex configuration of a broad complex tachycardia can only properly be judged from a 12-lead ECG. If the QRS complex is predominantly upright, or predominantly downward, in all the chest leads ('concordance' of the QRS complexes), ventricular tachycardia is likely. In the presence of a 'right bundle branch block' type complex (i.e. predominantly upright in V_1), a ventricular origin is likely if there is any of the following:

1. Left axis deviation
2. QRS complex shows a tall R wave and a deep S wave in V_6
3. In V_1 the initial R wave is greater than the secondary R wave $(R > R^1)$ – remember that in supraventricular rhythms, and right bundle branch block, the R^1 peak is always higher than the R peak.

In a broad complex tachycardia with a right bundle branch block pattern but none of the above features, a supraventricular origin is likely.

SUPRAVENTRICULAR TACHYCARDIA

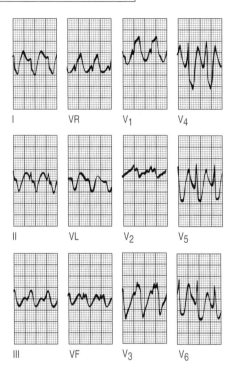

Note: Broad complex tachycardia
Right axis deviation
Right bundle branch block pattern
R waves of normal size in V_6
QRS complexes not predominantly upright in all leads
In V_1, R^1 is greater than R.

Conclusion: Probable supraventricular tachycardia with bundle branch block.

In the presence of a left bundle branch block pattern, i.e. QRS complexes predominantly downward in V_1, the 12-lead ECG is less helpful, but a ventricular origin of the tachycardia is likely if there is a QS pattern in V_6 (i.e. there is no R wave).

Fusion beats and capture beats

If an early beat can be found with a narrow QRS complex, it can be assumed that a wide complex tachycardia is ventricular in origin, because the narrow early beat demonstrates that the bundle branches will conduct supraventricular beats normally, even at high heart rates.

A 'fusion beat' is said to occur when the ventricles are activated simultaneously by a supraventricular and a ventricular impulse, so that a QRS complex with an intermediate pattern is seen.

A 'capture beat' occurs when the ventricles are activated by an impulse of supraventricular origin during a run of ventricular tachycardia.

VENTRICULAR TACHYCARDIA

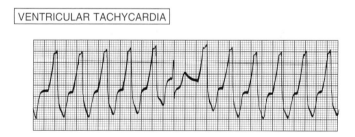

Note: A single early beat with a narrow QRS complex interrupts a broad complex tachycardia. The single beat (a 'capture' beat) must have a supraventricular origin, and by inference the broad complexes must have a ventricular origin.

Intra-atrial recording

Usually P waves cannot be seen in the ordinary ECG record during a broad complex tachycardia, but atrial activity can be demonstrated by passing a pacing catheter percutaneously into the right atrium, and recording from the catheter simultaneously with a surface ECG on a 2-channel recorder. In an intracardiac recording, the atrial activity is said to cause an 'A' wave and ventricular activity a 'V' wave.

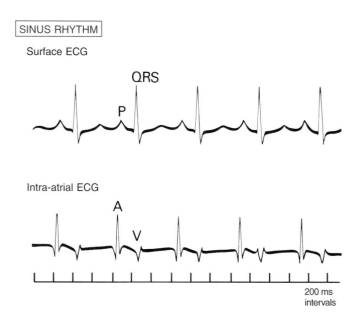

Note: Upper trace shows the normal surface ECG
Lower trace is recorded simultaneously from a pacing wire in the right atrium. The A wave (corresponding to the P wave in the surface ECG) appears much larger than the V wave (which corresponds to the QRS complex).

VENTRICULAR TACHYCARDIA

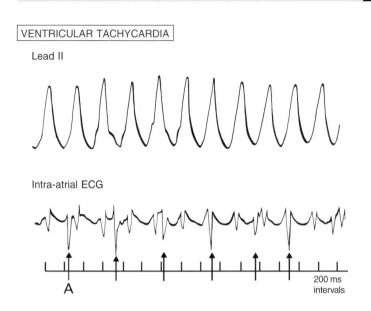

Lead II

Intra-atrial ECG

A

200 ms intervals

Note: In ventricular tachycardia, A waves can be seen in the right intra-atrial trace, at a slower rate and completely dissociated from the V waves. The V waves in an intra-atrial record always appear smaller than the A waves.

The presence of dissociated P waves proves that the rhythm has a ventricular origin. However, associated (1:1) P waves can occur in ventricular rhythms if the atria are activated in retrograde fashion up the His bundle.

Recording an intracardiac ECG is safe and simple, provided the appropriate equipment is available. However, it only becomes necessary when a patient has recurrent attacks of a broad complex tachycardia that are resistant to treatment.

Remember that in patients with myocardial infarction, a broad complex tachycardia is nearly always ventricular in origin. Remember also that a patient may withstand a ventricular tachycardia reasonably well for a while, and that it is not safe to assume that a rhythm must have a supraventricular origin because the patient looks well.

Polymorphic ventricular tachycardia and ventricular fibrillation

Ventricular tachycardia with a rate of over 200 per minute is often irregular and is associated with variation in the shape of the QRS complexes: this used to be called ventricular 'flutter', but is now called 'polymorphic ventricular tachycardia'.

POLYMORPHIC VENTRICULAR TACHYCARDIA

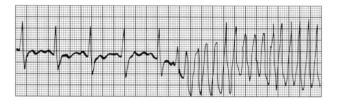

Note: Five sinus beats are followed by ventricular tachycardia at 300 per minute, with variation in the QRS complex configuration.

Polymorphic ventricular tachycardia has much the same effect as, and usually degenerates to, ventricular fibrillation.

VENTRICULAR FIBRILLATION

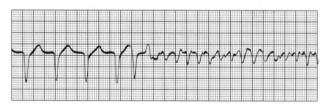

Note: The T wave of the fourth sinus beat is interrupted by a ventricular extrasystole (the R on T phenomenon). This is followed by the chaotic trace of ventricular fibrillation.

BRADYCARDIAS IN PATIENTS WITH SYMPTOMS

In this chapter we are primarily concerned with arrhythmias that cause symptoms; rhythms that are mainly of physiological interest are discussed in Chapter 6. This separation is, however, artificial, for whether or not an arrhythmia causes symptoms depends to some extent on how frequently it occurs.

The sick sinus syndrome

Supraventricular escape rhythms that occur intermittently are often asymptomatic, and are described in Chapter 6. They characterize the 'sick sinus syndrome', a condition in which abnormal SA node function may be associated with other abnormalities in the conducting system. The abnormal rhythms seen in the sick sinus syndrome (more properly called 'sinoatrial disease') include:

- Unexplained or inappropriate bradycardia
- Sudden changes in sinus rate
- Sinus pauses (sinoatrial arrest or exit block)
- Atrial standstill ('silent atrium')
- Atrioventricular junctional escape
- Atrial tachycardia associated with junctional escape
- Junctional tachycardia
- Atrial fibrillation with slow ventricular response
- Prolonged pauses after premature atrial beats.

Disordered SA node function can be familial or congenital, and can occur in ischaemic, rheumatic, hypertensive or infiltrative cardiac disease, but it is frequently idiopathic. The patient may be asymptomatic, but bradycardias can cause symptoms of heart failure and dizziness, and because atrial and junctional tachycardias often occur the patient may present with palpitations. The combination of sick sinus syndrome and tachycardias is sometimes called the 'bradycardia-tachycardia syndrome'. Rhythms that may be seen in this syndrome include 'sinus pauses' (sinus arrest and sinoatrial block) (see Ch. 6) and also atrial standstill (the 'silent atrium'). This is a common presentation, and the rhythm is maintained by junctional escape beats.

SICK SINUS SYNDROME

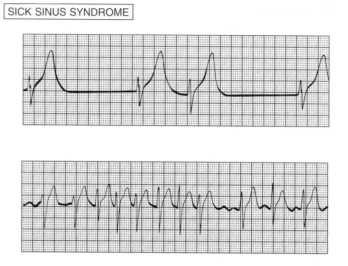

Note: Upper trace shows a 'silent atrium' with irregular junctional escape beats. With this rhythm the patient was asymptomatic, but he had episodes of junctional tachycardia (lower trace) which caused him to complain of palpitations. In the lower trace, junctional tachycardia is followed by a period of sinus rhythm.

The prognosis of patients with the sick sinus syndrome depends on the underlying disease, and patients with an idiopathic condition do well.

Atrioventricular block

Atrioventricular (AV) block can complicate any cardiac disease. It is common, and usually temporary, in acute myocardial infarction. Chronic heart block, particularly in elderly people, is usually a manifestation of fibrotic degeneration of the conducting system rather than of ischaemic heart disease.

First degree block and second degree block of the Wenckebach and Mobitz Type 2 varieties are asymptomatic. While they are indicators of heart disease and are of physiological interest, they are not in themselves clinically important (see Ch. 6). Second degree AV block with 2:1 atrioventricular conduction may cause symptoms if the ventricular rate is low enough.

Complete, or third degree, atrioventricular block can be asymptomatic or may cause heart failure. If the ventricular rate falls below a critical level the patient may lose consciousness in a Stokes-Adams attack.

COMPLETE BLOCK AND STOKES-ADAMS ATTACK

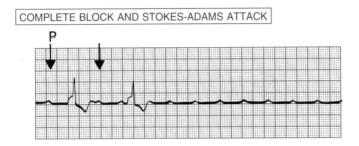

Note: After two complexes ventricular activity ceases, leaving only P waves. After a few seconds the patient lost consciousness in a Stokes-Adams attack.

The ECG in patients with pacemakers

Patients with bradycardias may be treated by the insertion of a temporary or permanent pacemaker. Occasionally the electrode that connects the pulse generator ('the battery') to the heart is sewn onto the epicardium. Usually, however, a 'wire' is inserted via a vein in the neck, through the right atrium and tricuspid valve, so that the tip of the electrode comes into contact with the endocardium of the right ventricle. In some patients two electrodes may be inserted, to allow stimulation of both the right atrium and the right ventricle.

Right ventricular stimulation maintains cardiac function because excitation spreads through the Purkinje system to the left ventricle. The rhythm is thus 'ventricular' in origin and the ECG shows a broad and abnormal QRS complex with an abnormal T wave. The electrical discharge of the pacemaker is recorded as a 'pacing spike' immediately before the QRS complex.

PACED RHYTHM

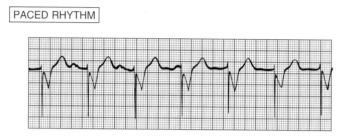

Note: The pacemaker stimulus causes a well-defined brief spike (often not seen as well as in this record), and this is followed immediately by a broad 'ventricular' QRS complex.

Early pacemakers were 'fixed rate', which meant that they produced pacing impulses at a constant frequency, independent of any spontaneous cardiac activity. The patient's own rhythm and that of the pacemaker could therefore compete.

FIXED RATE PACING

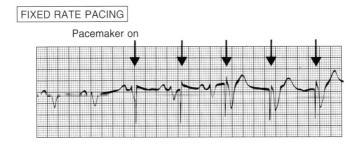

Note: After two sinus beats the pacemaker is switched on. The first pacing spike coincides with a QRS complex and the second with the T wave of a sinus beat: neither impulse stimulates the ventricle. A third pacing spike interrupts the T wave of a sinus beat, but the ventricles are stimulated and two further paced beats follow. The arrival of a pacemaker impulse on a T wave could precipitate ventricular fibrillation, but did not do so in this case.

All pacemakers are now of the 'demand' type, which means that they sense any spontaneous ventricular depolarization and this inhibits the pacemaker. For example, if the pacemaker is set at a demand rate of 60 per minute, it will delay for 1 second after any spontaneous heartbeat – this means that the heart rate will never fall below 60 per minute, but the rate may exceed this if spontaneous depolarization occurs more frequently.

'DEMAND' PACING

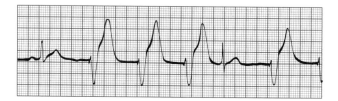

Note: After a sinus beat there is no cardiac activity for 920 ms.
The pacemaker is then activated at its pre-set rate of 70
per minute. After four paced beats, a single sinus beat
inhibits the pacemaker but after a further pause of 920 ms
the pacemaker is again activated.

Most modern pacemakers are 'programmable', which means
that their rate and some other characteristics of the impulses they
produce can be changed by an external 'programmer' after the
pacemaker has been inserted. 'Dual chamber' (right atrial and right
ventricular) pacemakers allow 'sequential' pacing of the atrium and
ventricle, so that the atrial contribution to cardiac output is
maintained. Some of these pacemakers automatically adjust their
rate to the physiological needs of the patient.

WHAT TO DO

What to do when an arrhythmia is suspected

24-hour (ambulatory) ECG monitoring

The only way to be certain that a patient's symptoms are due to
an arrhythmia is to record an ECG at the time they occur. When
symptoms are intermittent and infrequent, this can be extremely
difficult.

If the patient has symptoms at some time during most days it is
certainly worth recording the ECG continuously on a portable tape
recorder, while the patient carries on with his or her normal
activities. This is called 'ambulatory' or 'Holter' monitoring, after the

inventor of the initial recorder. Making and analysing these records is expensive in terms of technician time, and they are seldom helpful if the patient has symptoms less than once in every 2 or 3 weeks. For patients with infrequent attacks, cardiac 'event recorders' may be more useful: these are patient-activated, and store only brief sections of an ECG record.

If a patient records the presence of symptoms at a time when the ECG shows an arrhythmia, it is safe to assume that the symptoms and the arrhythmia are related. The following records were all obtained from patients who complained of palpitations or syncope, but who were in sinus rhythm at the time when they were examined, and their resting ECGs were normal.

24-H RECORD: SUPRAVENTRICULAR EXTRASYSTOLES

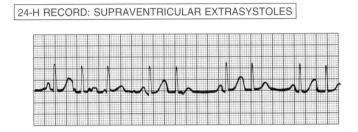

Note: Frequent supraventricular extrasystoles, recorded at the time when the patient had palpitations.

Occasionally a 24-hour ECG recording may show multiple abnormalities, and the rhythm associated with a major attack of symptoms may be recorded.

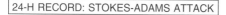

24-H RECORD: STOKES-ADAMS ATTACK

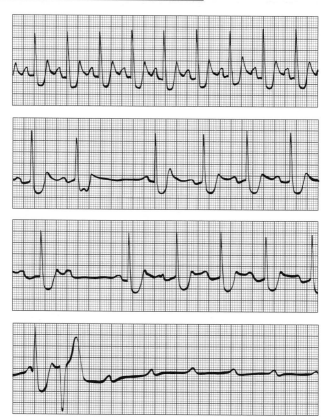

Note: Top strip shows sinus rhythm with normal AV conduction
Second strip shows sinoatrial block and third strip shows
second degree block – both these were asymptomatic.
Bottom strip shows a ventricular extrasystole followed by
complete heart block with ventricular standstill. The patient
lost consciousness due to this Stokes-Adams attack.

If the patient has no symptoms during the time the record is being made and the ECG shows sinus rhythm throughout, the investigation is unhelpful and a decision on whether to repeat it depends on clinical judgement. When the patient's story is highly suggestive of an arrhythmia, it may be justifiable to make repeated 24-hour records.

THREE 24-H RECORDS FROM ONE PATIENT

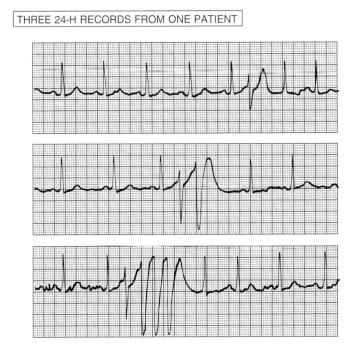

Note: Samples from three separate 24-hour records made at weekly intervals

Top strip shows sinus rhythm

Second record shows a couplet (pair) of ventricular extrasystoles (no symptoms noted)

Third record shows a short run of ventricular tachycardia, which corresponded to the patient's complaint of palpitations.

When the 24-hour ECG shows some arrhythmias which are not accompanied by symptoms, it is very difficult to be certain of their significance.

Table 2.5 shows the arrhythmias that were detected during two 24-hour periods in a group of 86 volunteers who were apparently completely free of heart disease. This study shows that supposedly dangerous arrhythmias such as ventricular tachycardia can occur and pass unnoticed in apparently healthy people.

Table 2.5 Arrhythmias observed during 48 hours of ambulatory recording in 86 healthy subjects aged 16–65 (from Clarke et al 1976 Lancet 2: 508–510).

Ventricular extrasystoles		63
(including: multifocal	13	
bigeminy	13	
R on T	3)	
Ventricular tachycardia		2
Supraventricular tachycardia		4
Junctional escape		8
Second degree block		2

Ventricular extrasystoles are so common that they can clearly be ignored, although epidemiological evidence suggests that in large groups of patients they can be crude 'markers' of heart disease. A few couplets of extrasystoles on a 24-hour record can also be accepted as being within the normal range.

24-H RECORD

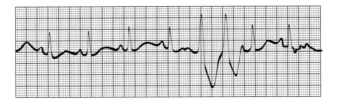

Note: Sinus rhythm with a couplet of ventricular extrasystoles – no associated symptoms.

Frequent couplets of ventricular extrasystoles, however, probably do indicate heart disease. If the patient complains of palpitations but has none at the time of recording even though the record shows frequent couplets, the occurrence of ventricular tachycardia must be suspected and either the record must be repeated or prophylactic treatment given.

24-H RECORD

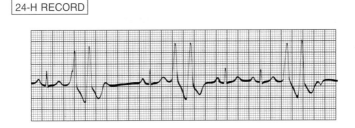

Note: Sinus rhythm with frequent couplets of ventricular extrasystoles.

When ventricular extrasystoles occur in runs of three or more the term 'salvoes' is sometimes used, but three or more ventricular extrasystoles together are usually considered to constitute 'sustained' ventricular tachycardia.

24-H RECORD

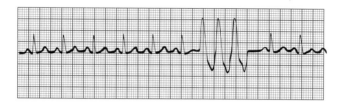

Note: Sinus rhythm with a short run of ventricular tachycardia.

Although even repeated short runs of ventricular tachycardia may not cause symptoms and may be seen in healthy people, they cannot be regarded as insignificant in patients with palpitations or syncope.

24-H RECORD

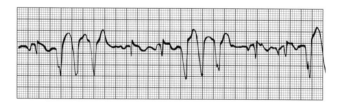

Note: Every two sinus beats are followed by a short run of ventricular tachycardia.

The progression from the asymptomatic and insignificant occasional couplet of ventricular extrasystoles to frequent short runs of ventricular tachycardia is gradual, and there is no certain point at which an arrhythmia that does not correspond with symptoms can be described as definitely significant. It can therefore be very difficult to know when to begin to treat an individual patient.

Patients who die suddenly while 24-hour ECG records are being made are usually found to have had ventricular fibrillation.

SUDDEN DEATH

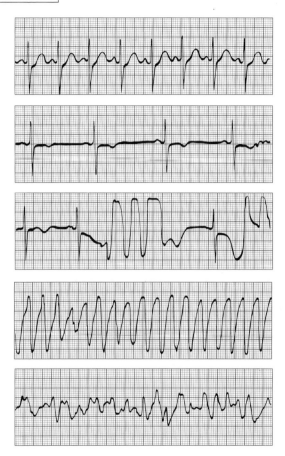

Note: First strip shows sinus rhythm. Sinus bradycardia develops, with inversion of the T waves suggesting ischaemia. Short runs of ventricular tachycardia lead to polymorphic ventricular tachycardia and then to ventricular fibrillation.

Precipitation of arrhythmias

Arrhythmias are sometimes precipitated by exercise, and if the patient's history suggests that this is so then treadmill testing may be helpful. Attempts to provoke an arrhythmia by exercise should, however, only be made when full resuscitation facilities are available.

PRECIPITATION OF AN ARRHYTHMIA

Rest

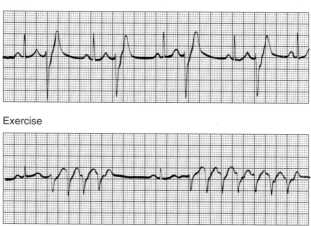

Exercise

Note: At rest the ECG shows frequent ventricular extrasystoles During exercise ventricular tachycardia occurs.

If the patient complains of syncopal attacks, particularly on movement of the head, it is worth pressing the carotid sinus in the neck to see whether the patient has carotid sinus hypersensitivity. Complete sinoatrial node inhibition may be induced, sometimes with unpleasant escape arrhythmias.

CAROTID SINUS HYPERSENSITIVITY

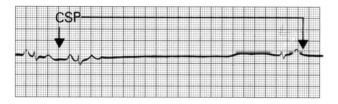

Note: Carotid sinus pressure causes cessation of all cardiac activity due to excessive vagal activity.

What to do when an arrhythmia is recorded

The first problem is to decide whether the arrhythmia has a cause that can or should be treated. The most common cause of arrhythmias is acute myocardial infarction, when any arrhythmia may arise. This is particularly likely after thrombolytic therapy, but the arrhythmias become progressively less common after the first 24 hours following the infarction. In some diseases arrhythmias are characteristic: for example, atrial fibrillation is part of the natural history of chronic rheumatic heart disease, and it is also common in alcoholic cardiomyopathy. In old people, thyrotoxicosis may present with atrial fibrillation but few other symptoms. Several drugs – notably digoxin and the tricyclic antidepressants – cause arrhythmias, and it is important to remember that the 'class I' anti-arrhythmic agents (e.g. quinidine, disopyramide, flecainide), and the 'class III' agents (e.g. amiodarone, sotalol), can also at times precipitate ventricular tachycardia.

The second problem is to decide whether the arrhythmia itself needs treatment. In general, arrhythmias that cause symptoms, or cause hypotension or signs of heart failure, must be treated. Those that have no effect can often be left untreated, but some arrhythmias are likely to cause problems unless treated: for example, a rapid and sustained supraventricular or ventricular tachycardia needs urgent treatment however well the patient appears to be, because deterioration is inevitable.

Since arrhythmias are most commonly encountered in patients with acute myocardial infarction, their management can be considered from this viewpoint – but in fact the principles are the same, whatever the patient's underlying disease. There are many anti-arrhythmic drugs, and all arrhythmias can be treated in more than one way. It is best, however, to use a limited number of drugs in a consistent way so as to gain experience with them. What follows is a simple and safe therapeutic policy, based on a few drugs.

Principles of arrhythmia management

1. Any arrhythmia causing significant symptoms or a haemodymamic disturbance must be treated immediately.
2. All anti-arrhythmic drugs should be considered as cardiac depressants and some can actually induce arrhythmias. The use of multiple agents should be avoided.
3. Electrical treatment (cardioversion for tachycardias, pacing for bradycardias) should be used in preference to drug therapy when there is marked haemodynamic impairment.

Management of cardiac arrest

The treatment of an individual patient will depend on the particular kind of arrhythmia involved.

Remember: Airway
                            Breathing
                            Cardiac massage

As soon as possible:
                            Intubate
                            Set up i.v. access

Ventricular fibrillation or pulseless ventricular tachycardia

1. Precordial thump
2. DC shock of 200 J
3. If unsuccessful, repeat DC shock of 200 J
4. If unsuccessful, DC shock of 360 J
5. If unsuccessful, give adrenaline 1 mg i.v.
6. 10 CPR (cardiopulmonary resuscitation) sequences (5 compressions:1 ventilation)
7. DC shock of 360 J
8. DC shock of 360 J
9. DC shock of 360 J
10. If unsuccessful, repeat:
11. After three loops, give lignocaine 100 mg i.v. and repeat loops.

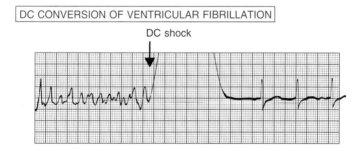

DC CONVERSION OF VENTRICULAR FIBRILLATION

DC shock

Note: Ventricular fibrillation (VF) is abolished by a DC shock, and a supraventricular rhythm (probably sinus in origin) immediately takes control of the heart.

It is not necessary to give routine anti-arrhythmic therapy after successful treatment of a first episode of VF.

Asystole

1. Precordial thump
2. If in any doubt about whether the arrhythmia is fine VF or asystole, treat as fine VF in the first instance

For asystole:

3. Adrenaline 1 mg i.v.
4. 10 CPR sequences (5 compressions:1 ventilation)
5. Atropine 3 mg i.v. (once only)
6. If unsuccessful, repeat steps 3 and 4:

7. After three loops, give adrenaline 5 mg i.v.
8. Successful correction of documented asystole should be followed by insertion of a temporary pacemaker.

Electromechanical dissociation (EMD)

EMD is characterized by QRS complexes without a palpable pulse. Consider specific therapy for the possible causes of EMD which are as follows:
- hypovolaemia
- pneumothorax
- cardiac tamponade (often due to cardiac rupture)
- pulmonary embolism
- drug overdoses
- electrolyte imbalance.

The general treatment of EMD (to be followed when no specific treatment is indicated) is:

1. Adrenaline 1 mg i.v.
2. 10 CPR sequences (5 compressions:1 ventilation)
3. If unsuccessful, repeat:

Remember that if an i.v. line cannot be established, you can give double or triple doses of adrenaline and atropine down an endotracheal tube.

Prolonged resuscitation

During any prolonged resuscitation, consider sodium bicarbonate 8.4% 50 ml i.v., taking blood gas results into account.

Post-resuscitation checks

- Arterial blood gas concentrations
- Electrolyte levels
- Chest X-ray
- ECG.

Management of other arrhythmias

Extrasystoles

Supraventricular: no treatment – if the patient has symptoms, explanation and reassurance.
Ventricular: usually no treatment, though treatment may be considered:

1. When ventricular extrasystoles (VEs) are so frequent that cardiac output is impaired
2. When there is a frequent R on T phenomenon
3. When the patient complains of an irregular heartbeat but reassurance and an explanation prove ineffective.

Three VEs together should be considered as ventricular tachycardia. The treatment of VEs is as for ventricular tachycardia.

Carotid sinus pressure in the management of tachycardias

The first step in the treatment of any tachycardia is carotid sinus pressure (CSP).

In sinus rhythm, carotid sinus pressure will cause transient lowering of the heart rate. This may be useful in identifying the true origin of the rhythm when there is doubt.

CSP AND SINUS RHYTHM

Without CSP

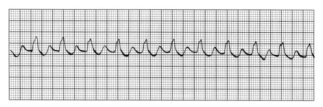

With CSP

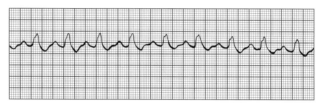

Note: Upper trace shows a broad complex tachycardia, and it is not obvious whether the biphasic deflection before the QRS complex represents a T wave or a T wave followed by a P wave. Lower record shows the effect of carotid sinus pressure. The rate falls and P waves are obvious.

In atrial flutter, atrioventricular conduction is blocked so that the ventricular rate falls. The atrial activity becomes obvious, which helps to identify the rhythm. Carotid sinus pressure seldom converts atrial flutter to sinus rhythm.

CSP AND ATRIAL FLUTTER

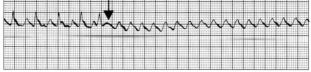

Note: Carotid sinus pressure increases the block at the AV node. Ventricular activity is completely suppressed and 'flutter' waves are obvious. Carotid sinus pressure can cause prolonged ventricular standstill, and can produce a syncopal attack.

In atrial tachycardia and junctional tachycardia, carotid sinus pressure may restore sinus rhythm.

CSP AND JUNCTIONAL TACHYCARDIA

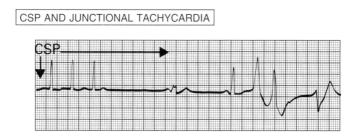

Note: Carotid sinus pressure reverts junctional tachycardia to sinus rhythm, but in this case multifocal ventricular extrasystoles occurred. Carotid sinus pressure should only be applied while the ECG is being monitored.

In atrial fibrillation and ventricular tachycardia, carotid sinus pressure has no effect. In the case of these, or any other rhythms, drug therapy may be needed.

Supraventricular tachycardias

Sinus tachycardia

Sinus tachycardia is a response to pain, anxiety, heart failure, hypovolaemia, thyrotoxicosis, anaemia, pregnancy, CO_2 retention, phaeochromocytoma or treatment with drugs which stimulate beta-adrenergic receptors. It is the primary cause which should be treated, not the sinus tachycardia itself.

Atrioventricular re-entry (junctional) tachycardia

The following treatment is suggested:

1. Carotid sinus massage.
2. Adenosine 3 mg i.v. bolus, followed if necessary after 2 mins by a further 6 mg adenosine and, if necessary after a further 2 mins, by a further 12 mg. N.B. Adenosine has a very short half-life. Unwanted but transient effects include an asthmatic attack, flushing, chest tightness and dizziness.
3. Verapamil 5–10 mg i.v., or atenolol 2.5 mg i.v. repeated at 5 minute intervals to a total of 10 mg. N.B. These two drugs should not be administered together, and verapamil should not be given to patients receiving a beta-blocker. The unwanted effects of verapamil may be reversed by calcium gluconate.
4. DC shock.

Second-line drugs (for use when initial treatment is unsuccessful) include digoxin, disopyramide, and amiodarone.

As prophylaxis for paroxysmal junctional tachycardia, try:

- atenolol
- verapamil
- disopyramide
- amiodarone.

Atrial tachycardia

This may be due to digoxin toxicity. Treat as for junctional tachycardia.

Atrial fibrillation and flutter
If the ventricular rate is less than 80 per minute, no treatment is needed. For immediate control of a rapid ventricular rate give one of:

- digoxin 250 μg i.v. slow injection, at 30 minute intervals to a total of 1 mg
- atenolol 2.5 mg i.v. repeated at 5 minute intervals to a total of 10 mg
- amiodarone (dose as for ventricular tachycardia, see below).

N.B. Amiodarone can potentiate digitalis effect. If cardioversion is needed in a digitalized patient, begin with very low energy shocks.

Conversion to sinus rhythm by drugs
Atrial fibrillation (AF) can seldom be converted to sinus rhythm by drugs. Atrial flutter may be converted by i.v. administration of sotalol, flecainide or disopyramide, but DC cardioversion is usually necessary.

Persistent fibrillation and flutter
Most patients who develop AF after a myocardial infarction will revert to sinus rhythm, but AF is a bad prognostic sign. Atrial flutter can be difficult to control, and cardioversion or atrial overdrive pacing may be needed.

For routine digitalization, digoxin orally, 500 μg initially, is followed by 250 μg thrice daily for 2 days. The maintenance dose of digoxin depends on the patient's renal function: 125–250 μg daily is usually adequate; old people and those with renal failure may need only 62.5 μg daily. N.B. Hypokalaemia potentiates the effects of digoxin.

Prevention of paroxysmal atrial fibrillation
Digoxin will not prevent attacks of paroxysmal atrial fibrillation, but the continuous use of one of the following may do so, at least for some months, or even years:

- verapamil
- sotalol
- flecainide
- disopyramide
- amiodarone.

In very resistant cases, electrical destruction (ablation) of the AV node can be used to cause complete heart block, and a permanent pacemaker is then inserted.

Ventricular tachycardia (VT)

VT is a broad complex tachycardia, occurring with a heart rate exceeding 120 per minute. It can be treated with one of:
- lignocaine 100 mg i.v., repeated twice at 5 minute intervals, followed by lignocaine infusion at 2–3 mg per minute (N.B. Lignocaine causes hypotension, drowsiness and sometimes fits)
- atenolol 2.5 mg i.v., repeated at 5 minute intervals to 10 mg
- flecainide 50–100 mg i.v.; for long-term treatment, 100 mg twice daily by mouth
- amiodarone 300 mg in 250 ml dextrose i.v. over 30 minutes, then 900 mg in 500 ml dextrose i.v. over 24 hours, followed by 200 mg thrice daily by mouth for 1 week, 200 mg twice daily for 1 week and 200 mg daily thereafter.

N.B. Amiodarone given i.v. must be given into a deep vein by long line. Overdose prolongs the QT interval and can cause tachycardia. Long-term treatment with amiodarone may cause skin pigmentation, photosensitive rashes, abnormalities of thyroid and liver function, drug deposits in the cornea, and occasionally pulmonary fibrosis.

Second-line drugs include disopyramide and mexilitine.

Recurrent episodes of ventricular tachycardia, particularly those that are drug-induced, can be terminated and sometimes prevented by pacing the right ventricle with a temporary pacemaker. In overdrive pacing, the rate is set faster than that of the VT and once the rhythm is captured by the pacemaker the rate can be slowed. Recurrent VT may be prevented by pacing at a rate of about 100 per minute, and this is particularly valuable in treating 'torsades' VT, when increasing the heart rate by pacing shortens the QT interval. In patients with recurrent VT, or those who have had more than one cardiac arrest with VF, an implanted defibrillator may be appropriate.

Patients with congenital long QT syndrome and paroxysmal VT are usually treated in the first instance with beta-blockers.

Wolff-Parkinson-White syndrome

In the paroxysmal tachycardia associated with the WPW syndrome, 're-entry' occurs, with excitation passing down the normal AV conduction pathway and back up the accessory pathway (see p. 264). Adenosine, digoxin, verapamil and lignocaine may increase conduction through an accessory pathway and block it in the AV node. This can be extremely dangerous if atrial fibrillation is associated with the pre-excitation syndrome, because ventricular fibrillation may occur. For this reason, these four drugs are not recommended for the treatment of pre-excitation tachycardias.

Drugs which slow conduction in the accessory pathway are:
- atenolol 5 mg i.v., repeated to 20 mg
- flecainide
- amiodarone.

For prophylaxis against paroxysmal arrhythmias, try one of:
- atenolol
- sotalol
- flecainide
- amiodarone.

The definitive, and now standard, treatment for tachycardias associated with the WPW syndrome is electrical ablation of the accessory pathway.

Bradycardias

Bradycardias must be treated if they are associated with hypotension, poor peripheral perfusion, or escape arrhythmias.

Any bradycardia can be treated with one of:
- atropine 600 µg i.v., repeated if necessary at 5 minute intervals to a total of 1.8 mg. N.B. Overdose causes tachycardia, hallucinations and urinary retention.
- isoprenaline 1–4 µg per minute (2 mg in 500 ml dextrose = 4 µg per ml). N.B. Overdose causes ventricular arrhythmias which can be difficult to treat. An isoprenaline infusion should only be used while preparations are made for pacing.

Temporary pacing in patients with acute myocardial infarction

Pacing should be *performed* under the following circumstances:
- complete block with ventricular rate below 50 per minute
- complete block with anterior infarction
- any persistent bradycardia needing an isoprenaline infusion
- bifascicular block plus first degree block.

Pacing should be *considered* in the case of:
- any complete block
- second degree block with heart rate less than 50 per minute
- bundle branch block plus first degree block
- evidence of increasing block
- bradycardia with escape rhythms
- drug-induced tachy-arrhythmias.

On the following pages are two complete ECGs from patients with arrhythmias, together with reports and interpretations.

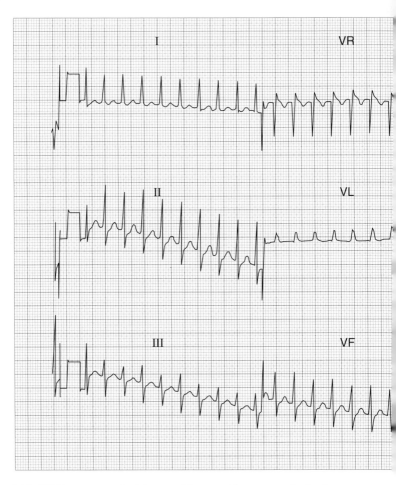

This ECG was recorded from a 30-year-old woman who had suffered occasional episodes of palpitations for 15 years, and was finally examined when she had symptoms.
The ECG shows:

- Regular, narrow complex tachycardia with a rate of 200 per minute
- No P waves can be seen
- Normal cardiac axis

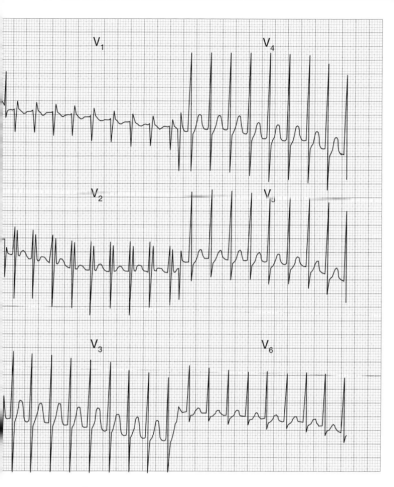

- RSR¹ pattern in leads V_1–V_2, but QRS complex duration is normal
- Normal ST segments and T waves.

Interpretation:

Junctional tachycardia. There is a 'partial RBBB' pattern in the V leads, but this is unlikely to be significant.

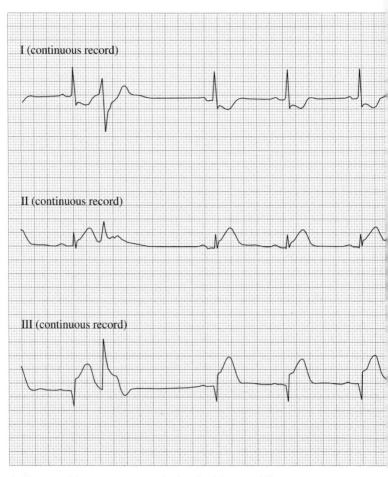

A 50-year-old man was seen in the Accident and Emergency Department complaining of chest pain. He collapsed while his ECG was being recorded, and no pulse could be felt.
The ECG shows:

- Sinus rhythm, with ventricular extrasystoles
- One extrasystole falls on the peak of the T wave of the preceding sinus beat (R on T phenomenon), and this is followed by ventricular fibrillation

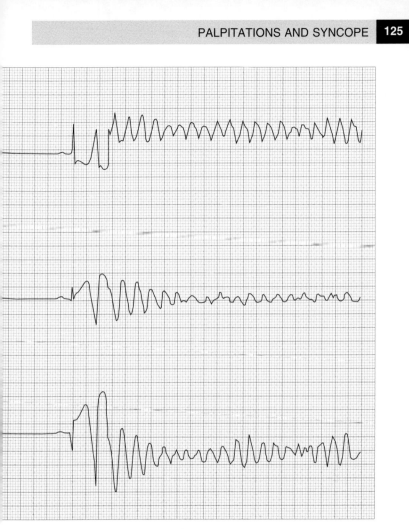

- A small Q wave in lead III
- Raised ST segments in leads II and III.

Interpretation:

Only leads I, II and III are available, but the raised ST segments suggest an acute myocardial infarction

CHAPTER 3

The ECG in patients with chest pain

HISTORY AND EXAMINATION

There are many causes of chest pain (see Table 3.1). All the non-cardiac conditions can mimic a myocardial infarction, and the ECG can be extremely useful when making a diagnosis. However, the ECG is less important than the history and physical examination, because the ECG can be normal in the first few hours of a myocardial infarction.

Table 3.1 Causes of chest pain

Acute	Chronic or recurrent
Myocardial infarction	Angina
Pulmonary embolism	Nerve root pain
Pneumothorax	Muscular pain
Other causes of pleuritic pain	Oesophageal reflux
Pericarditis	Nonspecific pain
Aortic dissection	
Ruptured oesophagus	
Oesophagitis	
Collapsed vertebra	

Acute chest pain

The pain of myocardial infarction is typically in the centre of the front of the chest, and it may radiate to the neck, jaw, teeth, arms or back. It is often severe and is then associated with sweating and sometimes vomiting. However, the pain can be mild or even, occasionally, absent.

The pain of a large central pulmonary embolus can be similar to that of myocardial infarction, but breathlessness and dizziness are usually also present. A peripheral pulmonary embolus will cause pleuritic pain and haemoptysis, and pleuritic pain due to embolism, infection or pneumothorax is usually easy to identify from the effect on respiration and coughing.

Pericardial pain is usually worse lying flat, and is relieved by sitting up and leaning forward; it may be affected by inspiration.

The pain of aortic dissection is often described by the patient as 'tearing' (as opposed to the 'crushing' pain of myocardial infarction), and it is typically felt mainly in the back.

Oesophageal rupture is always preceded by vomiting, and other oesophageal pain is usually associated with food and typically becomes worse on lying down.

Pain due to spinal disease can be identified from the effects of movement and position.

In all these conditions, the physical examination may be dominated by the effects of the pain itself: the patient may be anxious, often restless, and cold and sweaty. He or she will usually have a sinus tachycardia. The blood pressure is obviously important but diagnostically not necessarily helpful, because it can be low due to failure of the heart as a pump, or high due to intense peripheral vasoconstriction.

Each condition that causes chest pain may be associated with specific physical signs that are virtually diagnostic, but these may be absent and this is particularly likely in the early stages of the illness.

In myocardial infarction there may be pulmonary oedema and the jugular venous pressure may be elevated; there may be a third or fourth heart sound at the cardiac apex.

A large central pulmonary embolus will usually cause cyanosis and elevation of the jugular venous pressure, but there will be no added sounds in the lungs.

Pleuritic pain of any cause, and also pericarditis, will be associated with a friction rub.

Aortic dissection may cause the appearance of aortic valve regurgitation, and peripheral pulses may be lost. If blood flows back to the pericardium, there may be a pericardial friction rub.

Vertebral collapse usually causes local tenderness.

Oesophageal rupture causes few specific signs, and is a very easy diagnosis to miss.

As usual in medicine, the history is more helpful in the diagnosis of chest pain than is the physical examination, and both are more important than the ECG in the early stages of the patient's illness.

Chronic chest pain

The most common causes of chronic or intermittent chest pain are angina (pain due to temporary cardiac ischaemia) and musculoskeletal pain. An accurate diagnosis depends very much on the history: central crushing chest pain that radiates to the neck, jaw, teeth or arm, and which is predictably induced by exercise and relieved by rest, is likely to be angina. Typically, angina is worse in cold or windy weather, or during exercise after a meal; it is induced by sexual intercourse and also by excitement or emotional stress. Angina is often accompanied by breathlessness.

Pain that has similar characteristics to angina, but which is not closely related to exercise, may be due to spasm of the coronary arteries – but much more often, such pain is 'non-specific chest pain'. This sort of pain is common in young and in middle-aged men. It is usually felt in the left of the chest and may radiate to the left arm. It commonly occurs after exercise, or at the end of a busy day, and it may last an hour or more. Although it may apparently be induced by emotional stress, it is never caused by sexual intercourse.

Although angina is most often due to coronary artery disease, it is important to remember that it may be due to an arrhythmia, hypertension, valve disease (especially aortic valve disease), a cardiomyopathy, or anaemia. It is, therefore, important to exclude these possibilities by physical examination. Coronary artery disease itself causes no physical abnormalities, but a previous infarction may cause an enlarged heart, heart failure and perhaps mitral regurgitation. The signs of peripheral vascular disease may provide circumstantial evidence of the presence of coronary disease.

Non-specific chest pain causes no helpful abnormal signs, though chest wall tenderness may be present.

THE ECG IN PATIENTS WITH CHEST PAIN

Only after a full history has been taken and a careful physical examination has been made is it sensible to look at the ECG. The ECG is helpful when it shows unequivocal abnormalities, but when it does not it is much safer to rely on the patient's history and physical signs when making the diagnosis.

In the diagnosis of the various conditions that cause chest pain, the ECG is most useful in the case of myocardial infarction. It is helpful in the diagnosis of angina, if a recording can be made when the patient has pain. It may provide confirmatory evidence of a pulmonary embolus, but the changes are seldom diagnostic, and although in pericarditis there may be ECG abnormalities, these are usually nonspecific and the ECG is not often very helpful.

THE ECG IN PATIENTS WITH MYOCARDIAL INFARCTION

It must be remembered that 'myocardial infarction' is really a pathological diagnosis, and if the patient survives there is no certain way of confirming that an infarction has occurred. There has been much disagreement about a clinical definition for myocardial infarction: when the history is clear, the ECG is unequivocal, and the serum enzymes that correlate with infarction (creatine kinase and lactate dehydrogenase) rise to twice their upper limit of normal, then there will be little doubt that infarction has occurred. However, it can be difficult to be certain that ECG changes are new and a marginal rise of serum enzymes is common in patients with suspected infarction. It is best only to label the patient as having had a 'definite' infarction when both the ECG *and* the serum enzymes show unequivocal changes; when one of these is doubtful, 'probable infarction' is an acceptable diagnosis. When neither is unequivocal, 'possible infarction' is a reasonable label, but this merges into 'ischaemic disease without evidence of infarction'. 'Chest pain, ?cause' is an entirely proper diagnosis when the ECG and serum enzymes are normal but the patient is admitted with chest pain for which no diagnosis can be made.

The development of ECG changes in infarction

The most important function of the ECG in patients with suspected myocardial infarction is to monitor the rhythm of the heart so that significant arrhythmias (especially ventricular fibrillation) can be treated rapidly. Rhythm problems have been considered in Chapter 2, and here we need to think about the ECG as a diagnostic aid.

It is essential to remember that in the first hour or more after the onset of chest pain due to myocardial infarction, the ECG can remain normal. Up to 20% of patients admitted to hospital with what subsequently proves to be myocardial infarction may show little or no abnormality in their first ECG. However, fully developed infarct patterns can arise very quickly indeed. Typically, first the ST segment becomes raised, then Q waves appear, and finally the ST segment returns to the baseline and the T waves become inverted.

DEVELOPMENT OF INFERIOR MYOCARDIAL INFARCTION

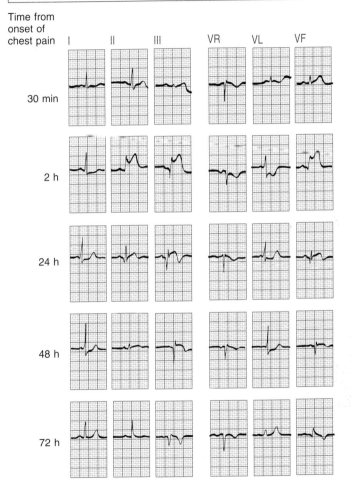

| Time from onset of chest pain | I | II | III | VR | VL | VF |

Note: Initial ECG shows inverted T wave in VL, but no other abnormality ST segment then becomes elevated in the inferior leads Q waves develop, the ST segment returns to normal and the T waves become inverted.

Because there is a very variable speed of development of the ECG changes in myocardial infarction, it is difficult to decide from a single ECG when the infarction occurred. Serial changes in two or three records taken during the first 3 days after a suspected infarction are the most convincing evidence. Although classically the raised ST segment returns to the ECG baseline, this does not always occur, and particularly following anterior infarction a raised ST segment may persist indefinitely. This is sometimes associated with a left ventricular aneurysm, but it is not a reliable way of making this diagnosis.

OLD ANTERIOR INFARCTION: LEFT VENTRICULAR ANEURYSM

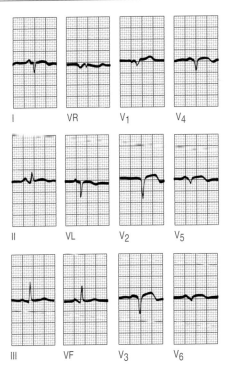

I VR V₁ V₄

II VL V₂ V₅

III VF V₃ V₆

Note: This patient had had an anterior infarction several months previously, but the ST segments in leads V₂–V₅ remained elevated. In this case, a left ventricular aneurysm was present.

Once present, Q waves usually persist, but when the infarction is small, Q waves can disappear over a period of months as the infarction heals, and the ECG can return to normal. When this happens the patient's prognosis is very good.

Anterior infarction

The part of the heart that is infarcted is indicated by the ECG leads that show the infarct pattern. Thus an infarction of the anterior wall of the left ventricle and the septum causes changes in the leads that 'look at' the front of the heart, V_2–V_5.

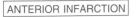

ANTERIOR INFARCTION

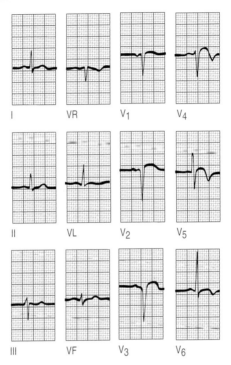

Note: The ECG is normal in the limb leads, apart from T wave flattening in VL

There is a Q wave in V_1–V_3, and only a rudimentary R wave in V_4

The ST segment is elevated in V_2–V_5

The T wave is inverted in V_4–V_6

The elevated ST segments suggest that the infarction is acute, but the presence of Q waves suggests that it occurred at least an hour or two previously.

An old anterior infarction may be associated with very small R waves in V_1–V_4/V_5 rather than with Q waves: this is sometimes called 'loss of R wave progression' (see p. 17).

Antero-lateral infarction

When the infarction affects the anterior and lateral walls of the left ventricle, the changes occur in the anterior leads and also in the leads that 'look at' the lateral aspect of the heart, namely I, VL, and V_5–V_6.

ACUTE ANTERO-LATERAL INFARCTION

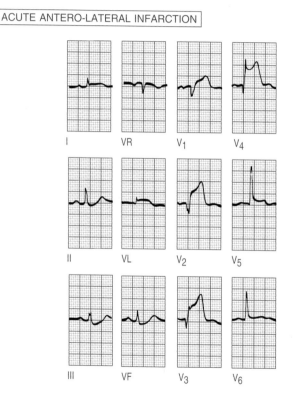

Note: Raised ST segments in I, VL, and V_1–V_6
Q waves in V_2–V_4.

Inferior infarction

When the inferior wall of the left ventricle is affected, the ECG changes are seen in the 'inferior' leads, III and VF, and sometimes also in lead II.

INFERIOR INFARCTION

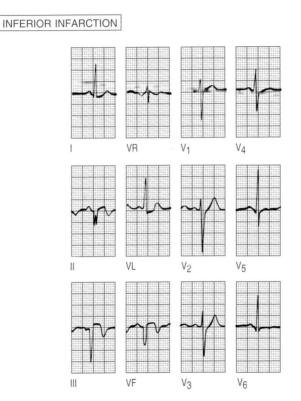

Note: Q waves with raised ST segments and inverted T waves in leads II, III and VF
The chest leads show a normal appearance.

Anterior and inferior infarction

Infarction of both the anterior and inferior walls of the left ventricle causes changes in the anterior and the inferior leads.

ANTERIOR AND INFERIOR INFARCTION

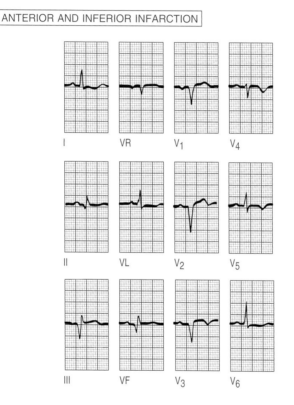

Note: Q waves in III and VF indicate old inferior infarction
Q waves in V_2–V_3 and a rudimentary R wave in V_4, plus inverted T waves in VL and V_3–V_6, indicate an anterior infarction and lateral ischaemia.

Posterior infarction

It is possible to 'look at' the back of the heart by placing the V lead on the back of the left side of the chest, but this is not done routinely because it is inconvenient and the complexes recorded are often small.

An infarction of the posterior wall of the left ventricle can, however, be detected in the ordinary 12-lead ECG because it causes a dominant R wave in lead V_1. The shape of the QRS complex recorded in V_1 depends on the balance of electrical forces reaching the ECG electrode. Normally the right ventricle is being depolarized towards this electrode, so causing an upward movement (an R wave) in the record; and at the same time, the posterior wall of the left ventricle is being depolarized, the wave of excitation moving away from the electrode and so causing a downward movement (an S wave) in the record. The left ventricle is more muscular than the right and exerts a greater influence on the ECG, so in V_1 the QRS complex is predominantly downward (i.e. there is a small R wave and a deep S wave). In a posterior infarction, the rearward-moving forces are lost, so V_1 'sees' the unopposed forward-moving depolarization of the right ventricle, and records a predominantly upright QRS complex.

POSTERIOR INFARCTION

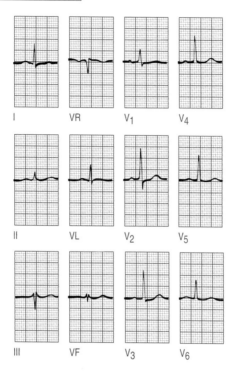

Note: The limb leads are normal
In V_1 there is a dominant R wave
There are no other changes to suggest right ventricular hypertrophy.

A posterior infarction is sometimes called a 'true posterior' infarction, because in old terminology what is now called 'inferior' used to be called 'posterior'. The dominant R wave of a (true) posterior infarction causes an ECG appearance very similar to that of right ventricular hypertrophy, but there is no accompanying right axis deviation. It is the patient's history and the lack of right ventricular hypertrophy on physical examination that are most important in making the diagnosis.

Postero-lateral infarction

Infarction can affect both the posterior and lateral walls of the left ventricle.

POSTERO-LATERAL INFARCTION

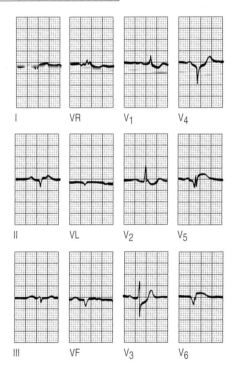

I VR V_1 V_4

II VL V_2 V_5

III VF V_3 V_6

Note: Sinus rhythm
Dominant R wave in V_1
Q waves in I, VL, V_5–V_6
Elevated ST segments in V_5–V_6.

Right ventricular infarction

Inferior infarction is sometimes associated with infarction of the right ventricle. Clinically, this is suspected in a patient with an inferior infarct when the lungs are clear but the jugular venous pressure is elevated. The ECG will show a raised ST segment in leads recorded from the right side of the chest, in positions corresponding to those on the left side. These leads are called V_2R, V_3R, V_4R etc.

Recurrent infarction

When a patient has a second myocardial infarction, the ECG will show whether a different part of the heart has been damaged. The next four records show how useful sequential recordings can be.

1st RECORD: INFERIOR INFARCTION

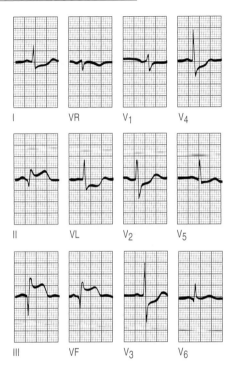

I   VR   V₁   V₄

II   VL   V₂   V₅

III   VF   V₃   V₆

Note: This record was taken from a patient with recent onset of chest pain, and shows an acute inferior infarction with Q waves and raised ST segments in leads II, III and VF. There is horizontal ST segment depression in leads V_2–V_5. This is sometimes called 'reciprocal' depression, and it represents ischaemia in the territory not affected by the infarction. Evidence of disease in two main territories (in this case inferior and anterior) indicates a poor prognosis.

A few hours later, the patient had more pain:

2nd RECORD: ATRIAL FIBRILLATION, INFERIOR AND
ANTERIOR INFARCTION

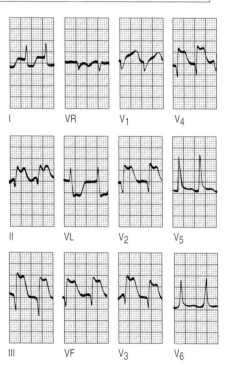

| I | VR | V₁ | V₄ |

I   VR   V₁   V₄

II   VL   V₂   V₅

III   VF   V₃   V₆

Note: This record shows atrial fibrillation with a rapid ventricular
rate. The chest leads now show raised ST segments,
suggesting an acute anterior infarction.

The patient recovered and sinus rhythm was restored. The next record was taken 24 h after the second:

3rd RECORD: SINUS RHYTHM, INFERIOR AND ANTERIOR INFARCTION

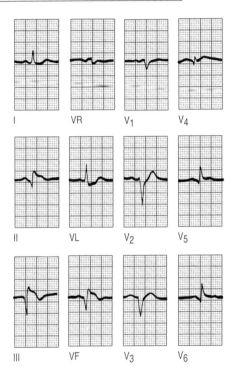

| I | VR | V₁ | V₄ |

| II | VL | V₂ | V₅ |

| III | VF | V₃ | V₆ |

Note: Sinus rhythm. The ECG now shows a loss of R waves in V_2–V_4, and a diagnosis of both inferior and anterior infarction can be made.

A few weeks later, when the patient was clinically well, the ECG showed evidence of an old inferior and an old anterior infarction:

4th RECORD: OLD INFERIOR AND ANTERIOR INFARCTION

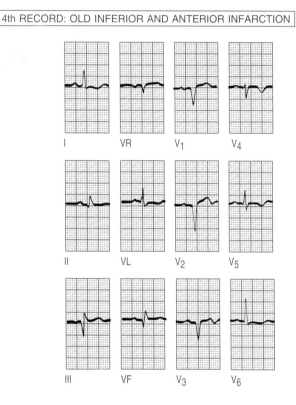

I   VR   V₁   V₄

II   VL   V₂   V₅

III   VF   V₃   V₆

Note: In the inferior leads, III and VF, the Q waves persist but the T waves have become upright
Q waves in V_2–V_3 and inverted T waves in V_3–V_6 show an old anterior infarction.

Infarction of the interventricular septum

A large infarction of the interventricular septum can cause damage to both bundle branches, and the ECG pattern of combined right and left bundle branch block is, of course, that of complete heart block. The QRS complex is then wide and the T wave is abnormal, and no infarct pattern can be detected. Similarly, if an infarction causes left bundle branch block it is not possible to detect infarct changes on the ECG record.

LEFT BUNDLE BRANCH BLOCK

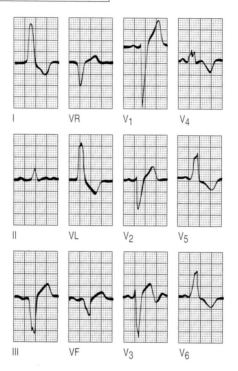

Note: Sinus rhythm

Broad QRS complexes with a notched R wave in V_5–V_6 show LBBB

Inverted T waves are associated with LBBB

Any ischaemia is masked by this pattern.

However, block of only the anterior fascicle of the left bundle branch does not obscure the infarction pattern, and the pattern of marked left axis deviation (left anterior hemiblock – see Ch. 6) and an anterior infarction pattern shows that part of the septum has been damaged.

LEFT ANTERIOR HEMIBLOCK WITH ANTERIOR INFARCTION

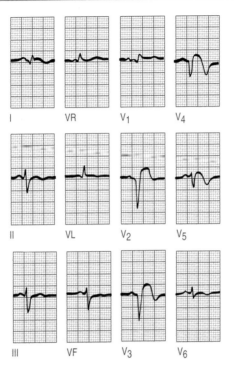

I	VR	V₁	V₄
II	VL	V₂	V₅
III	VF	V₃	V₆

Note: Sinus rhythm
Deep S waves in leads II and III show left axis deviation
(left anterior hemiblock)
Anterior chest leads show elevated ST segments and
inverted T waves, due to anterior infarction.

With right bundle branch block due to septal infarction, it is sometimes possible to be confident that an infarction has occurred.

RBBB WITH ANTERIOR INFARCTION

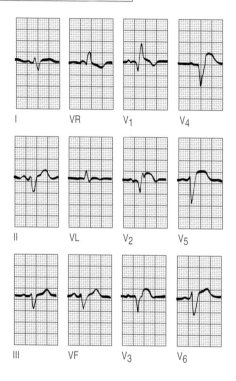

Note: Sinus rhythm

Left axis deviation

QRS complex duration greater than 120 ms

RSR^1 pattern in V$_1$ shows RBBB

Combination of left axis deviation and RBBB indicates bifascicular block (see p. 257)

Q waves in V$_2$–V$_4$ with raised ST segments show anterior infarction.

Non-Q wave infarction

When the infarction does not involve the whole thickness of the ventricular wall, no electrical 'window' will be formed, so there will be no Q waves. There will, however, be an abnormality of repolarization that leads to inversion of the T waves. This pattern is most commonly seen in the anterior and lateral leads. It is sometimes called 'subendocardial infarction', but the pathological changes seen in heart muscle after a myocardial infarction often do not fit neatly into 'subendocardial' or 'full thickness' patterns. Compared to patients with Q wave infarctions, those with non-Q wave infarctions have a high incidence of reinfarction during the following 3 months, but thereafter their fatality rates are similar.

NON-Q WAVE INFARCTION

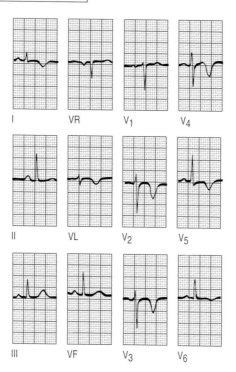

I VR V₁ V₄

II VL V₂ V₅

III VF V₃ V₆

Note: No Q waves are present, but the T waves are inverted in I, VL, and V_2–V_6 due to antero-lateral non-Q wave infarction.

THE ECG IN PATIENTS WITH ANGINA

The patient who has angina but who has not had myocardial infarction will usually have a normal ECG while he or she is free of pain. The ECG will become abnormal when the patient has angina, and the characteristic change is horizontal depression of the ST segments.

ST segment depression is not, however, caused only by ischaemia: for example, it is also seen in the ECGs of patients treated with digoxin (when the ST segment slopes downwards, rather than being depressed horizontally as in ischaemia) or quinidine.

ISCHAEMIA

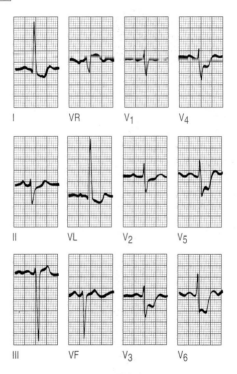

Note: Sinus rhythm with left axis deviation
Horizontal or downsloping depression of the ST segments in leads I, VL and V_3–V_6 indicates ischaemia.

The diagnosis of ischaemic pain can be made whatever the precipitating cause. For example, when pain occurs during a spontaneous episode of a paroxysmal attack of supraventricular tachycardia, depression of the ST segments indicates ischaemia.

ISCHAEMIA DURING JUNCTIONAL TACHYCARDIA

Note: Junctional tachycardia (no P waves and narrow QRS complexes) at 170 per minute
ST segment depression in I, II, and V_3–V_6 indicates ischaemia.

Angina can occur at rest, due to spasm of the coronary arteries. This is accompanied by elevation rather than depression of the ST segments. The ECG appearance is similar to that of an acute myocardial infarction, but the ST segment returns to normal as the pain settles. This ECG appearance was first described by Prinzmetal, and it is sometimes called 'variant' angina.

PRINZMETAL'S VARIANT ANGINA

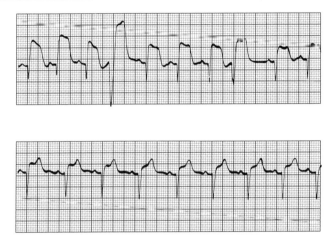

Note: The two strips form a continuous record
Initially the ST segment is raised; the fourth beat is probably a ventricular extrasystole
The ST segment quickly becomes normal.

In most patients with intermittent chest pain, however, it will be necessary to stress the patient in some way to induce angina, and the safest procedure for this is the exercise test.

EXERCISE TESTING

Although any form of exercise that induces pain should produce ischaemic changes in the ECG, it is best to use a reproducible test that patients find reasonably easy to perform, and to use carefully graded increments of exercise. The use of non-standard tests means that their results may be difficult to interpret, and that repeated tests in the same patient cannot be compared meaningfully. It is important to remember that exercise testing provides much useful information in addition to causing changes in the ST segment of the ECG. Things to look for during an exercise test include:

1. The patient's attitude to exercise
2. The reason for exercise limitation:
   - chest pain
   - breathlessness
   - claudication
   - fatigue
   - musculo-skeletal problems
3. The pumping capability of the heart
   - maximum heart rate achieved
   - maximum rise in blood pressure
4. Physical fitness
   - workload at which maximum heart rate is achieved
   - duration of tachycardia following exercise
5. Ischaemic changes in the ECG
6. Exercise-induced arrhythmias.

Reproducible exercise testing needs either a bicycle ergometer or a treadmill. In either case, the exercise should begin at a low level that the patient finds easy, and should be made progressively more difficult. On a bicycle, the pedal speed should be kept constant and the workload increased in 25 watt steps. On a treadmill, both the slope and the speed can be changed and the protocol evolved by Bruce (Table 3.2) is the one most commonly used.

Table 3.2 Bruce protocol for exercise testing using a treadmill, 3 minutes at each stage

	Low level			Ordinary level				
Stage	01	02	03	1	2	3	4	5
Speed (km/h)	2.7	2.7	2.7	2.7	4.0	5.5	6.8	8.0
Slope (degrees)	0	1.3	2.6	4.3	5.4	6.3	7.2	8.1

Alternatively, a Naughton protocol can be used: this involves a much slower increase of workload (Table 3.3).

Table 3.3 Modified Naughton protocol, 2 minutes at each stage

Stage	0	1	2	3	4	5	6	7	8	9	10
Speed (km/h)	1.6	2.4	3.2	3.2	3.2	4.8	4.8	4.8	4.8	5.5	5.5
Slope (degrees)	0	0	2	4	6	4.3	5.7	7.1	8.5	8	9

A 12-lead ECG, the heart rate and the blood pressure should be recorded at the end of each exercise period.

The maximum heart rate and blood pressure are in some ways more important than the maximum workload achieved, because the latter is markedly influenced by physical fitness.

Indications for discontinuing the test are:

1. At the request of the patient, because of pain, breathlessness, fatigue or dizziness.
2. If the systolic blood pressure begins to fall. Normally, systolic pressure will rise progressively with increasing exercise levels, but in any subject a point will be reached at which systolic pressure reaches a plateau and then starts to fall. A fall of 10 mmHg is an indication that the heart is not pumping effectively and the test should be stopped; if it is continued, the patient will become dizzy and may fall. In healthy subjects, a fall in systolic pressure is seen only at high workloads, but in patients with severe heart disease the systolic pressure may fail to rise on exercise. The amount of exercise the patient can carry out before the systolic pressure falls is thus a useful indicator of the severity of any heart disease.
3. It is conventional to discontinue the test if the heart rate increases to 80% of the predicted maximum for the patient's age: this maximum can be calculated in beats per minute by subtracting the patient's age in years from 220. Patients with severe heart disease will usually fail to attain 80% of their predicted maximum heart rate, and the peak heart rate is another useful indicator of the state of the patient's heart. It is,

of course, important to take note of any treatment the patient may be receiving, because a beta-blocker will prevent the normal increase in heart rate.

4. Exercise should be discontinued immediately if an arrhythmia occurs. The use of exercise testing to provoke arrhythmias is discussed in Chapter 2; many patients will have ventricular extrasystoles during exercise, and these can be ignored unless their frequency begins to rise, or a couplet of extrasystoles occurs.

5. The test should be stopped if the ST segment in any lead becomes depressed by 4 mm; 2 mm of horizontal depression in any lead is usually taken as indicating that a diagnosis of ischaemia can be made (a 'positive' test), and if the aim of the test is to confirm or refute a diagnosis of angina there is no point in continuing once this has occurred. It may, however, be useful to find out just how much a patient can do, and if this is the aim of the test it is not unreasonable to continue if the patient's symptoms are not severe.

The final report of the test should indicate the duration of exercise, the workload achieved, the maximum heart rate and systolic pressure, the reason for discontinuing the test, and a description of any arrhythmias or ST segment changes.

The record on the opposite page was obtained from a patient with a history suggesting angina, but whose ECG at rest was normal.

Note: Single complexes from each of leads V_3–V_6 at rest and at the end of four stages of exercise following the Bruce protocol. Stage 02 is a low level of exercise. With increasing exercise, the heart rate rises progressively but at the final stage the BP falls. There is progressive ischaemic ST segment depression in all leads, but especially in V_4.

EXERCISE TEST (BRUCE PROTOCOL)

Stage	Rest	02	1	2	3
Rate	95	123	131	148	168
BP	120/70	170/100	180/100	185/105	170/100

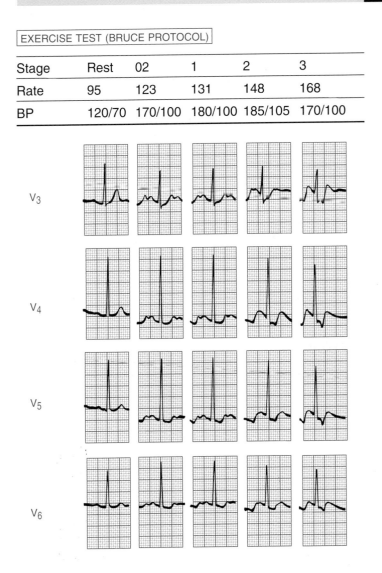

Ambulatory recording

An alternative to a treadmill test, although usually less satisfactory, is to look for ST segment depression in an ambulatory ECG tape recording. It is important that the recorder is of the correct sensitivity for this test to be reliable. Ambulatory recording is mainly of value in studying patients whose chest pain is not clearly related to exercise.

AMBULATORY RECORDING – ECG AT REST

No pain

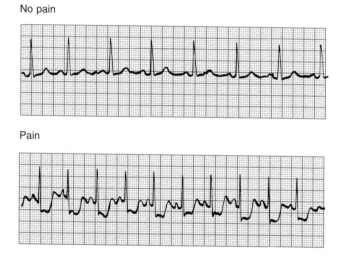

Pain

Note: Upper trace shows a normal ECG in V_4. During an episode of chest pain at rest, there is 4 mm ST segment depression.

Other ECG changes during exercise

It is important to differentiate between ischaemic changes in the ST segment and upward-sloping ST segment depression. The junction between the S wave and the ST segment is sometimes called the 'J point' (not to be confused with the 'J wave' seen in hypothermia), and upward-sloping ST segment depression is sometimes called 'J point depression'. This is a non-specific change.

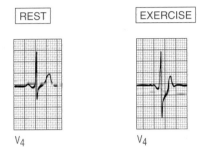

Note: Left-hand complex is from V_4 at rest. Right-hand complex shows upward-sloping ST segment during exercise, with depression of the 'J point'. This is a normal result.

T wave inversion alone can be non-specific, and may simply be related to hyperventilation. When a T wave that is inverted at rest becomes upright during exercise, ischaemia is probably present.

Elevation rather than depression of the ST segment during exercise may be due to abnormalities of movement of the left ventricular wall, as occur in ventricular aneurysms.

Exercise often induces ventricular extrasystoles, but these are not in themselves useful indicators of ischaemia.

Dangers of exercise testing

Because exercise testing can induce arrhythmias, it must be supervised by a doctor.

The next three records were obtained before, during, and immediately after an exercise test.

REST

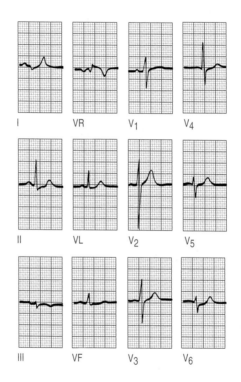

EXERCISE

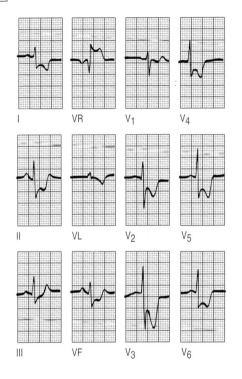

1 MINUTE AFTER EXERCISE

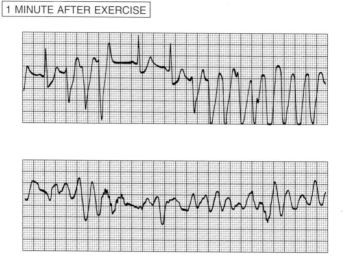

Note: The record at rest is normal
Exercise to the point at which the patient complained of chest pain caused marked horizontal ST segment depression (8 mm in V_3), with T wave inversion.
1 minute after exercise, there was a short run of VT, followed by two sinus beats, then a return to VT which rapidly decayed to VF. (Such a response is rare, but usually indicates severe coronary disease.)

The diagnostic accuracy of exercise testing

The value of exercise testing in detecting significant coronary disease depends on the sensitivity, specificity and predictive accuracy of the test. 'Sensitivity' is the chance that the test will detect the condition if it is present (i.e. it indicates the false negative rate) and 'specificity' is the chance that a positive result really indicates disease (i.e. it indicates the false positive rate). 'Predictive accuracy' takes both into account, but also depends on the prevalence of the disease in the population being studied. To take an extreme example, if the disease is rare, a test that has low sensitivity might miss all the patients who had the disease and a test with low specificity might give more false positive than real positive results.

In patients who have had a myocardial infarction and who therefore have coronary disease, different studies have given widely different results for the detection of multi-vessel coronary disease. This has possibly occurred because different exercise protocols were used, studying maximal or sub-maximal exercise, and different end-points were taken to indicate the end of the test. Roughly, however, an exercise test in such patients has a sensitivity of 65%, a specificity of 85% and a predictive accuracy of 80% for identifying those with disease of more than one coronary artery. An exercise test probably has greater predictive accuracy than this for detecting disease of the left main coronary artery, or severe three-vessel coronary disease, but even in patients with these conditions, exercise testing is by no means infallible.

In healthy people, the predictive accuracy of exercise testing for the later development of symptomatic coronary disease is about 20%.

Exercise testing is commonly used in post-infarction patients, to assess 'residual ischaemia' and in the hope that high-risk patients can be identified. The precise role of exercise testing in this situation is not clear, because results depend very much on the exercise protocol used and the period that has elapsed since the infarction. Although some early studies suggested that the development of ischaemia indicated a poor prognosis, later work showed that the prognosis was only poor if the left ventricle was so damaged that exercise induced only a poor response in terms of heart rate and blood pressure.

THE ECG IN PULMONARY EMBOLISM

Although the ECG can be helpful in making the diagnosis of pulmonary embolism, it is not to be relied upon because most patients with a pulmonary embolus will have no ECG abnormality other than a sinus tachycardia.

Pulmonary embolism causes problems for the right ventricle, and when multiple pulmonary emboli cause chronic pulmonary hypertension, the full range of possible changes due to right ventricular hypertrophy may be seen.

MULTIPLE PULMONARY EMBOLI

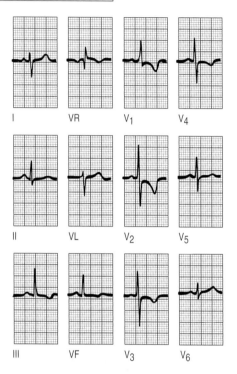

Note: Right axis deviation
Dominant R wave in V_1
Persistent S wave in V_6
Inverted T waves in V_1–V_4.

It is, however, most unusual for the full ECG appearance of right ventricular hypertrophy to be seen with an acute pulmonary embolus. This diagnosis is likely if the chest pain is associated with sinus tachycardia and any of the ECG changes mentioned in the notes beneath the record opposite.

PULMONARY EMBOLUS

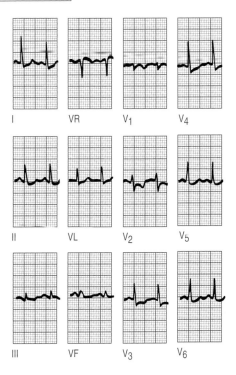

Note: Sinus tachycardia at 130 per min
Normal QRS complexes in V_1
T wave inversion in V_1–V_4.

The significance of minor abnormalities may only be apparent if they are seen to appear in comparison with a previously normal ECG, – for example, the appearance of right axis deviation may indicate pulmonary embolism.

? ACUTE PULMONARY EMBOLUS

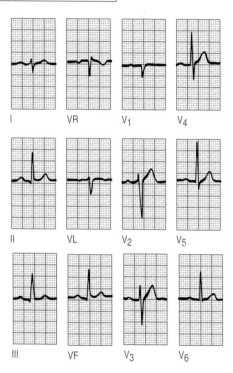

Note: Dominant S wave in lead I indicates right axis deviation. This could be normal, but it could also be the only ECG change due to a pulmonary embolus.

Another ECG pattern which could be within the normal range is T wave inversion in V_1–V_2. If, however, the T waves in these leads are initially upright but then become inverted, pulmonary embolism is likely – as is shown in the next two records.

NORMAL ECG

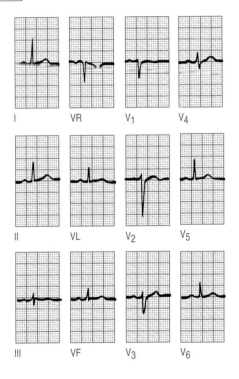

I	VR	V_1	V_4
II	VL	V_2	V_5
III	VF	V_3	V_6

2 DAYS LATER: PULMONARY EMBOLUS

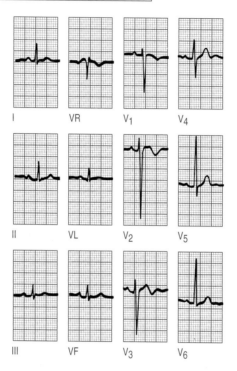

I   VR   V₁   V₄

II   VL   V₂   V₅

III   VF   V₃   V₆

Note: The first record is entirely normal. The second record,
which was made 2 days later after an episode of chest
pain, shows T wave inversion in V_1–V_2 and a biphasic T
wave in V_3. This record could be within normal limits, but in
comparison with the first it is clearly abnormal, and
indicates a pulmonary embolus. The change in height of
the QRS complex is not significant.

The combination of right axis deviation with a Q wave and an inverted T wave in lead III is said to be characteristic of pulmonary embolus, though it is by no means diagnostic.

PULMONARY EMBOLUS

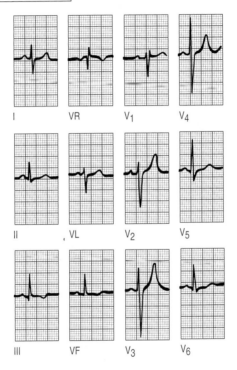

Note: 'S$_I$, Q$_{III}$, T$_{III}$' pattern of pulmonary embolus
The chest leads are normal.

Finally, acute pulmonary embolism may cause right bundle branch block, but this is frequently seen in patients who do not have a pulmonary embolus, so only the recorded appearance of this ECG abnormality is of much significance.

PULMONARY EMBOLUS

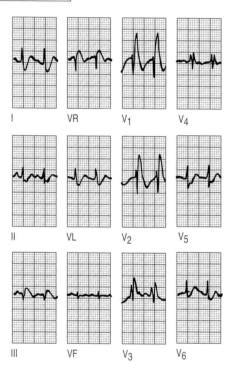

Note: Sinus tachycardia, rate 160 per minute
Right bundle branch block.

Pulmonary emboli can also cause supraventricular arrhythmias.
The possible ECG changes in pulmonary embolism may be
summarized as:

- Sinus tachycardia
- Right axis deviation
- Dominant R wave in V_1
- Inverted T wave in V_1–V_3 or V_4
- Right bundle branch block
- Q wave and inverted T wave in III
- Supraventricular arrhythmias.

THE ECG IN OTHER CAUSES OF CHEST PAIN

Pericarditis

Pericarditis may cause widespread ST segment/T wave changes.
Classically, the ST segment is elevated and the change resembles
acute myocardial infarction, with the difference that most leads are
affected and Q waves do not develop. This 'classical' ECG pattern
is, in fact, rare.

ACUTE PERICARDITIS

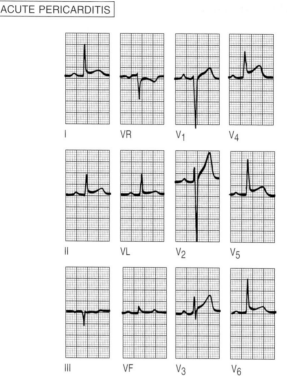

I   VR V_1 V_4

II   VL V_2 V_5

III   VF V_3 V_6

Note: Widespread ST segment elevation, concave upwards
No Q waves to suggest infarction.

Aortic stenosis

If a patient complains of chest pain that sounds like angina and the ECG shows left ventricular hypertrophy, it is important to remember that he or she may have severe aortic valve disease, and may need valve replacement urgently. Alternatively, the left ventricular hypertrophy could be the result of long-standing hypertension.

LEFT VENTRICULAR HYPERTROPHY

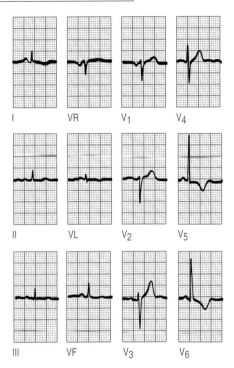

Note: Sinus rhythm with normal axis
Tall R waves in V_5–V_6
Inverted T waves in I, VL, and V_5–V_6 indicate left
ventricular hypertrophy.

Aortic dissection

In patients with aortic dissection the ECG may show the changes
of left ventricular hypertrophy if the patient has been hypertensive
(see Ch. 4), but in many patients the dissection results from
medial necrosis of the aorta without preceding hypertension, and

the ECG is then normal. If the dissection occludes a coronary artery, the ECG changes of an infarction may develop.

DIFFERENTIAL DIAGNOSIS OF ECG PATTERNS IN ISCHAEMIA

There are several situations in which ECG patterns can be confused with those of ischaemia or infarction: most of these involve abnormalities of the ST segment and T wave.

The ECG pattern in the Wolff-Parkinson-White syndrome can at first sight suggest a mistaken diagnosis of a non-Q wave infarction.

WOLFF-PARKINSON-WHITE SYNDROME

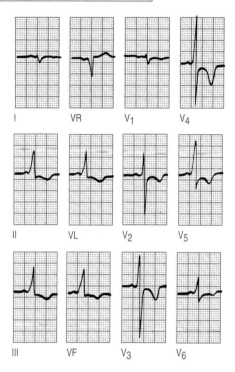

Note: Sinus rhythm, with a short PR interval and slurred upstroke of the R wave due to pre-excitation
The widespread T wave inversion is characteristic of WPW syndrome, and must not be mistaken for a non-Q wave infarction.

In hypertrophic cardiomyopathy (a condition that may present with ischaemic cardiac pain), the ECG may show widespread deep T wave inversion, resembling that of a non-Q wave infarction.

HYPERTROPHIC CARDIOMYOPATHY

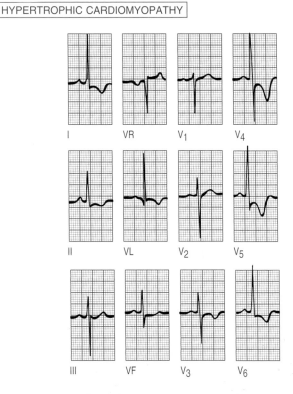

Note: Marked T wave inversion in the antero-lateral leads, giving an appearance more like ischaemia than left ventricular hypertrophy.

Table 3.4 summarizes some of the potential pitfalls in the diagnosis of the cause of chest pain.

Table 3.4 Pitfalls in the diagnosis of the cause of chest pain

Condition	ECG pattern	May be confused with
Normal record	Q waves in III but not VF T wave inversion in V_1–V_3 (especially in black people)	Inferior infarction Anterior infarction
Left ventricular hypertrophy	T wave inversion in lateral leads	Ischaemia
Right ventricular hypertrophy	Dominant R waves in V_1 Inverted T waves in V_1–V_3	Posterior infarction Anterior infarction
Wolff-Parkinson-White syndrome	Inverted T waves in V_2–V_5	Anterior infarction
Hypertrophic cardiomyopathy	T wave inversion in V_2–V_5	Anterior infarction
Subarachnoid haemorrhage	T wave inversion in any leads	Ischaemia
Digitalis effect	Downsloping ST segment depression or T wave inversion, especially in V_5–V_6	Ischaemia

WHAT TO DO

It is essential to remember that while the ECG can on occasions be extremely helpful in the diagnosis of chest pain, frequently it is not. The history, and to a lesser extent the physical examination, are far more important.

Acute chest pain suggesting myocardial infarction

If the history suggests that the patient has had a myocardial infarction, the aims of treatment are:

1. Pain relief
2. Getting the patient quickly to an ambulance or hospital where cardiac arrest can be properly managed should it occur
3. Making a more certain diagnosis
4. Instituting thrombolytic therapy, if there are no contraindications.

The risk of death is highest soon after the onset of symptoms, and thrombolytic treatment is most effective if given promptly. It is, therefore, essential to arrange admission to hospital as soon as possible, and for many patients it is better to summon an emergency ambulance than to seek help from their general practitioner.

The value of pre-hospital thrombolysis is debatable: the advantage of starting treatment a little earlier has to be set against the possibility of giving a thrombolytic agent to a patient with a peptic ulcer or dissecting aneurysm, and also against the risks of hypotension and bradycardia, which can be difficult to manage in an ambulance. Although extrasystoles and tachy-arrhythmias are common after thrombolysis, they are not particularly important.

To reduce the risk of treating patients inappropriately, it is customary to give thrombolytic treatment only to those whose ECG shows changes that are at least suggestive of an infarction. These changes are any of the following:

- ST segment elevation equal to or greater than 1 mm in two or more limb leads, or equal to or greater than 2 mm in two or more chest leads
- left bundle branch block, unless this is known to be of long standing.

Thrombolytic therapy is effective whichever site of infarction is indicated by the ECG. Right ventricular infarcts are treated in the same way as are left ventricular infarcts, except that vasodilators must be avoided in the treatment of right ventricular infarction; the left ventricle is often under-filled, and the administration of fluid (preferably with haemodynamic monitoring using a Swan-Ganz catheter) may be needed.

Old or equivocal ECG changes, or bundle branch block, do not provide sufficient indication for thrombolysis unless supported by measurements of cardiac enzyme levels.

The best-established thrombolytic regimen is:

1. Soluble aspirin 300 mg, chewed immediately

2. Streptokinase 1.5 million units, infused over 1.5 h
3. Heparin i.v. for 24 h.

The alternative thrombolytic agents rt-PA (alteplase) or RPA (reteplase) may possibly cause less adverse reactions than streptokinase, but these are seldom severe with any agent, and do not justify the high cost of these newer agents. These *are* indicated in patients who have previously been treated with streptokinase, in whom the presence of antibodies may make streptokinase less effective and at the same time may increase the risk of severe allergic reaction.

It is not clear whether a beta-blocker given i.v. has any effect if aspirin and streptokinase are being given. There is no evidence that the routine use of prophylactic anti-arrhythmic drugs is beneficial, and indeed it may be harmful.

Investigations for acute chest pain

In the majority of patients, detailed physical examination and the organization of investigations other than the ECG can be delayed until the pain has been completely relieved and thrombolytic therapy has been completed.

Chest X-rays are seldom helpful and unless a pneumothorax or some other cause of pleurisy, or a dissecting aneurysm, seem possible the patient should not be detained in the Accident and Emergency Department waiting for an X-ray examination. Chest X-rays taken using portable equipment are seldom helpful, and it is often best to wait until the patient is well enough to go to the Radiology Department.

Echocardiography is the investigation of choice if pericarditis is suspected, as most patients will have a pericardial effusion which is easily detected. Echocardiography may help in the diagnosis of an aortic dissection, but not reliably; computed tomography scanning is probably the investigation of choice, though this too can be very misleading.

Chronic chest pain

Chronic or intermittent chest pain must be investigated and treated as the history dictates. If angina seems likely but the resting ECG is normal, an exercise test may be useful in establishing the diagnosis and giving a rough indication of the severity of the angina. However, a stress test is not mandatory if the symptoms are mild.

The indications for coronary angiography are not clearly defined, and depend very much on the personal preference of individual physicians. Angiography is obviously essential if coronary artery bypass grafting or percutaneous transluminal coronary angioplasty is being considered, so patients still symptomatic despite maximum medical therapy need to be investigated. Angiography is also probably necessary in young people with a strongly positive exercise test at a low workload (say, 3 mm depression at Bruce Stage 2 or less), but opinion varies as to whether this threshold should be applied when the patient is medically treated or not. Practice in North America usually involves early angiography, while in the UK it is only performed in a small proportion of patients who are treated for angina.

A trial of sublingual glyceryl trinitrate 0.5 mg may help make the diagnosis of angina, and in such cases patients should then be encouraged to use the drug liberally and prophylactically. Beta-blockers are the first-line agents for preventing angina; all have much the same effect and a cardioselective agent such as atenolol 50–100 mg daily is best. If the patient is unable to take a beta-blocker (e.g. because of asthma), treatment should start with a calcium-channel blocker such as nifedipine 10–20 mg thrice daily or diltiazem 60–120 mg thrice daily. Beta-blockers and calcium-channel blockers can be combined, and a long-acting nitrate such as isosorbide mononitrate 20 mg twice daily can be added. 'Maximum medical therapy' for angina usually implies the simultaneous use of a drug of each of these types in the maximum dose that the patient can tolerate without suffering unpleasant side-effects.

The next four pages show the full ECG traces of two patients who were seen in an Accident and Emergency Department with chest pain.

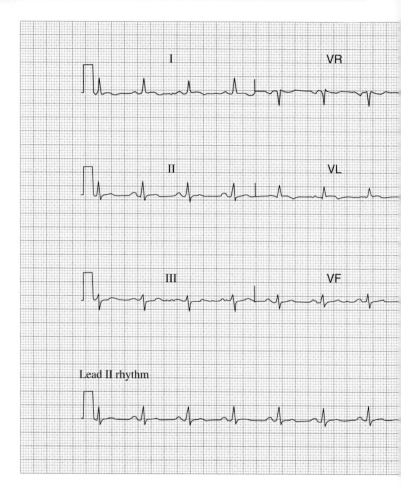

This ECG was recorded from a 55-year-old man who came to the Accident and Emergency Department complaining of severe central chest pain. There were no abnormal physical signs. The ECG shows:

- Sinus rhythm
- Normal cardiac axis
- Normal conducting intervals

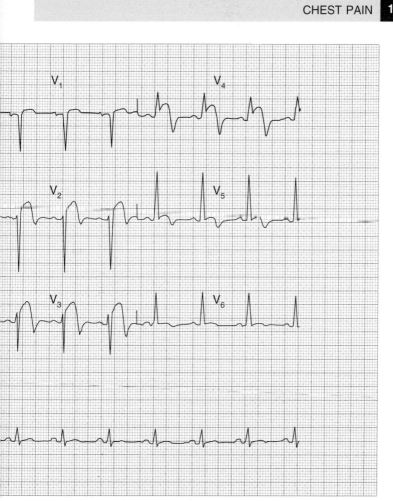

- Normal QRS complexes
- Raised ST segments in V_2–V_5
- Inverted T waves in VL and V_3–V_5.

Interpretation:

Acute anterior myocardial infarction.

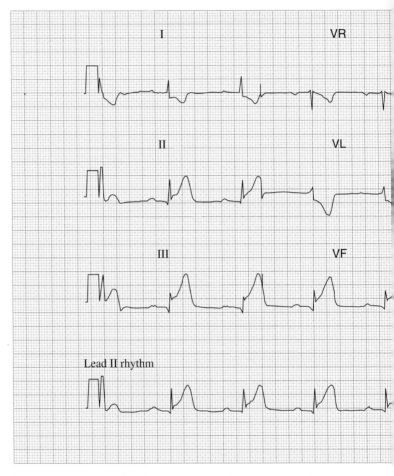

This ECG was recorded from a 60-year-old man who was seen in the Accident and Emergency Department, having had severe central chest pain for 2 hours.

The ECG shows:

- Sinus rhythm
- Normal cardiac axis
- Normal conducting intervals
- Small Q waves in leads III and VF

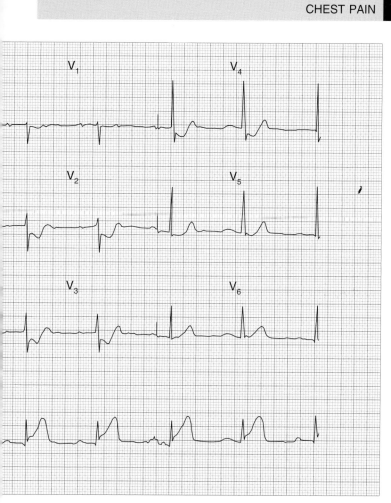

- Raised ST segments in leads II, III and VF
- Depressed ST segments in leads I, VL, V_2–V_4
- Inverted T waves in leads I and VL.

Interpretation:

Acute inferior myocardial infarction, with ST segment/T wave changes in the anterior and lateral leads, indicating ischaemia.

CHAPTER 4

The ECG in patients with breathlessness

HISTORY AND EXAMINATION

There are many cause of breathlessness (Table 4.1). Everyone is breathless at times, and people who are physically unfit or who are overweight will be more breathless than others.
Breathlessness can also result from anxiety, but when it is due to physical illness the important causes are anaemia, heart disease and lung disease; a combination of causes is common. The most important function of the history is to help to determine whether the patient does indeed have a physical illness and if so, which system is affected.

Breathlessness in heart disease is due either to increased lung stiffness as a result of pulmonary congestion, or to pulmonary oedema.

Pulmonary congestion occurs when the left atrial pressure is high, but is still lower than the oncotic pressure exerted by the plasma proteins. A high left atrial pressure occurs either when mitral stenosis impairs blood flow from the left atrium to the left ventricle, or when the left ventricle is failing and its filling pressure (the end-diastolic pressure) is high. The recognition of pulmonary congestion is less easy than that of pulmonary oedema, because it can be confused with chest disease causing right heart failure (cor pulmonale). In both, the patient may complain of orthopnoea: in heart failure, this is due to the return to the effective circulation of blood that was pooled in the legs, while in patients with chest disease (especially chronic obstructive airways disease) orthopnoea results from a need to use diaphragmatic respiration

Table 4.1 Causes of breathlessness

Physiological and psychological causes	Lack of fitness Obesity Pregnancy Locomotor diseases (including ankylosing spondylitis) Anxiety
Heart disease – left ventricular failure	Ischaemia Mitral regurgitation Aortic stenosis Aortic regurgitation Congenital disease Cardiomyopathy Arrhythmias
– high left atrial pressure	Mitral stenosis Atrial myxoma
Lung disease	Any interstitial lung disease, e.g. infection, tumour, infiltration Pulmonary embolism Pleural effusion Pneumothorax
Pericardial disease	Constrictive pericarditis
Anaemia	

more effectively. Both pulmonary congestion and lung disease can cause a diffuse wheeze. Both pulmonary congestion and cor pulmonale will be associated with signs of right heart failure. The diagnosis therefore depends on a positive identification, either in the history or on examination, of heart or lung disease.

When the haemodynamic pressure of blood within the pulmonary capillaries (which is the same as that in the pulmonary veins and left atrium) exceeds the oncotic pressure of plasma, fluid will leak into the alveoli and cause pulmonary oedema. The presence of pulmonary oedema is relatively easy to recognize from a history of orthopnoea (breathlessness on lying flat), severe breathlessness (especially with attacks at night) with wheeze, and a cough productive of frothy sputum, which may be pink or frankly blood-stained. Physical examination reveals fine crackles over the lung bases; there are usually other signs of heart failure such as a raised jugular venous pressure, ankle swelling, or hepatic distension; and the heart is usually large.

The main causes of heart failure are ischaemia, valve disease, hypertension, congenital defects, heart muscle disease, and arrhythmias. Ischaemia and arrhythmias can usually be suspected from the patient's symptoms and sometimes from the physical examination: the value of the ECG in diagnosing these conditions was considered in Chapters 2 and 3. Congenital disease will be suspected from the history and examination, and the presence of valve disease may be suspected if the patient gives a history of previous rheumatic fever. However, the diagnosis of valve disease, heart muscle disease and hypertension depends mainly on the physical examination. The value of the ECG in diagnosing these conditions is quite limited, and in general all it can do is provide information about the size of the four heart chambers.

The ECG also has only limited value in the diagnosis of respiratory disease. The diagnosis depends on a history of cough, wheeze and sputum production, and on the physical signs of lung disease. The ECG can only show whether lung disease has caused enlargement of the right atrium and right ventricle.

THE ECG IN DISORDERS AFFECTING THE LEFT SIDE OF THE HEART

The ECG in left atrial hypertrophy

Left atrial hypertrophy may be associated with left ventricular hypertrophy, but left atrial hypertrophy without left ventricular hypertrophy is virtually diagnostic of mitral stenosis. Mitral stenosis causes right ventricular hypertrophy, and this may be evident on the ECG record (see p. 201). ECG evidence of left atrial hypertrophy is, however, seldom helpful in assessing the severity of mitral valve disease. This is because most patients develop atrial fibrillation, and with the loss of P waves no information about the size of the left atrium is available.

When the heart is in sinus rhythm, left atrial hypertrophy causes a broad and sometimes bifid P wave, often best seen in lead II. Because this is characteristic of mitral stenosis, this P wave abnormality is sometimes called 'P mitrale'.

LEFT ATRIAL HYPERTROPHY

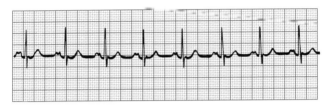

Note: Sinus rhythm
The P waves are broad and bifid (i.e. have two humps).

The ECG in left ventricular hypertrophy

Left ventricular hypertrophy may be caused by hypertension, aortic stenosis or incompetence, or mitral incompetence.

The ECG features of left ventricular hypertrophy are:
- an increased height of the QRS complex
- inverted T waves in the leads that 'look at' the left ventricle: I, VL, and V_5–V_6.

Left axis deviation is not uncommon, but it is due more to fibrosis than to the left ventricular hypertrophy itself.

Unfortunately, none of these features is an infallible indication of left ventricular size, and the following two records from patients with severe aortic stenosis illustrate the problem.

The first record, which was from a patient with congenital aortic stenosis with a pressure gradient across the valve of 80 mmHg (indicating severe stenosis), leaves no doubt about left ventricular hypertrophy.

LEFT VENTRICULAR HYPERTROPHY

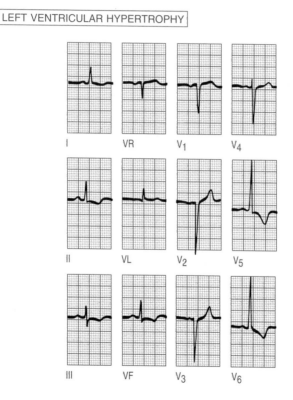

Note: Tall R wave in V_5–V_6 and a deep S wave in V_2
Inverted T waves in II, III, VF, V_5–V_6
The axis is normal.

This appearance is sometimes referred to as a 'left ventricular strain' pattern, but this is a meaningless term. The record was in fact made 8 years after an aortic valve replacement, when the patient was completely well and the left ventricle was certainly not under 'strain', but the ECG appearance of left ventricular hypertrophy had not changed as a result of the operation.

The second record came from another patient with severe aortic stenosis (with a pressure gradient of 85 mmHg across the valve), and this patient was breathless and needed valve replacement. The ECG was, however, entirely normal.

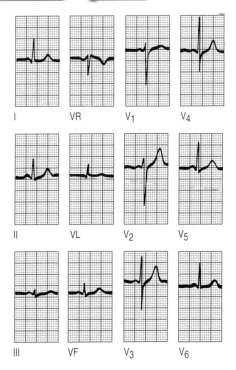

AORTIC STENOSIS: NORMAL RECORD

Note: No evidence of left ventricular hypertrophy
Normal-sized QRS complexes and upright T waves.

Between these two extremes, ECG evidence of left ventricular hypertrophy can be very variable. The normal maximum height of the R wave in lead V_5 or V_6, and also the normal maximum depth of the S wave in V_1 and V_2, are often set at 25 mm. The maximum height of the R wave in V_5 or V_6 plus the depth of the S wave in V_1 or V_2 is supposed in normal people to be less than 35 mm. However, these limits are frequently exceeded in the ECGs of young fit people, particularly if they are thin (Ch. 1). The next ECG record, however, came from an 18-year-old who had had an aortic valve replacement for the treatment of congenital aortic stenosis.

?LEFT VENTRICULAR HYPERTROPHY

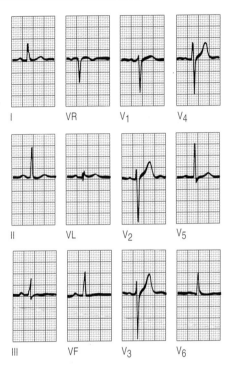

I   VR   V₁   V₄

II   VL   V₂   V₅

III   VF   V₃   V₆

V leads at half normal sensitivity

Note: Sinus rhythm, normal axis
The record looks entirely normal, but the chest leads were
recorded with a sensitivity of 0.5 cm representing 1 mV.
The 'true' height of the QRS complexes is thus twice that
recorded. The record shows LV hypertrophy by 'voltage'
criteria.

As we have seen (Ch. 1), minor left axis deviation occurs in the ECGs of normal people who are short and fat. Marked left axis deviation may be seen in patients with left ventricular hypertrophy, but it is really an indication of a conduction defect rather than of ventricular mass. Marked left axis deviation is due to failure of conduction through the anterior fascicle of the left bundle branch ('left anterior hemiblock'), and this can occur without any enlargement of the left ventricle.

The next ECG came from an asymptomatic patient whose heart was clinically normal.

LEFT ANTERIOR HEMIBLOCK

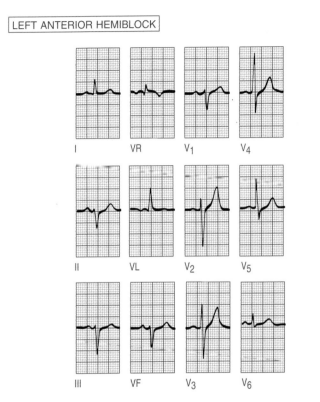

Note: Sinus rhythm

Marked left axis deviation, with a dominant S wave in leads II and III.

The combination of either tall complexes or left axis deviation with inverted T waves in the lateral leads makes a diagnosis of left ventricular hypertrophy likely. In any patient with valve disease, the appearance of ECG changes characteristic of left ventricular hypertrophy in serial recordings should be taken as evidence of deterioration. However, the T wave changes in the lateral leads can vary from time to time. The next record shows the chest leads in two records taken 6 months apart from an elderly patient with aortic valve disease.

LEFT VENTRICULAR HYPERTROPHY

First record (chest leads only)

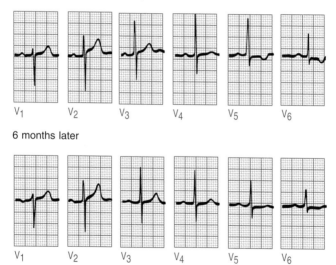

6 months later

Note: First record (chest leads only) shows T wave inversion in V_5–V_6. This is much less obvious in the second record.

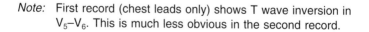

Lateral T wave inversion can result from ischaemia as well as from left ventricular hypertrophy, and the next record was from a patient with a myocardial infarction.

NON-Q WAVE INFARCTION

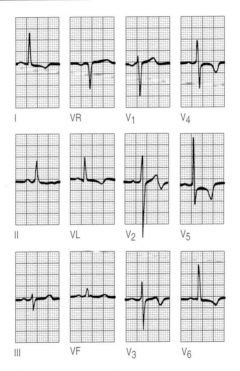

Note: Sinus rhythm, normal axis
Normal QRS complexes
T wave inversion in I, VL and V_2–V_6.

The presence of ischaemia rather than left ventricular hypertrophy should be suspected if any pathological Q waves are present; if T wave inversion is present in the 'septal' lead V_4; or if T wave inversion is more marked in V_3–V_5 than in V_6.

The ECG in patients with mitral valve prolapse

When mitral valve prolapse is severe, the ECG may show features of left ventricular hypertrophy, but in less severe cases there can be a variety of ECG changes which are often inconsistent. These changes include T wave inversion (often in leads II, III and VF but also in any of the anterior leads), ST segment changes that resemble ischaemia, and arrhythmias including ventricular extrasystoles and atrial fibrillation.

THE ECG IN DISORDERS AFFECTING THE RIGHT SIDE OF THE HEART

The ECG in right atrial hypertrophy

Right atrial hypertrophy causes tall and peaked P waves. There is, in fact, such variation within the normal range of P waves that the diagnosis of right atrial hypertrophy is difficult to make, but its presence can be inferred when peaked P waves are associated with the ECG changes of right ventricular hypertrophy. The changes of right atrial hypertrophy without those of right ventricular hypertrophy will usually only be seen in patients with tricuspid stenosis.

RIGHT ATRIAL HYPERTROPHY

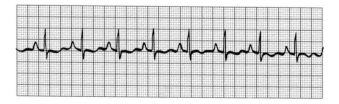

Note: Sinus rhythm
Peaked P waves, due to right atrial hypertrophy ('P pulmonale')
The T waves are inverted, but in a single lead it is not possible to see why.

The ECG in right ventricular hypertrophy

Right ventricular hypertrophy can be the result of chronic lung disease (e.g. chronic obstructive airways disease, bronchiectasis etc.), pulmonary embolism (especially when repeated episodes cause thromboembolic pulmonary hypertension), idiopathic pulmonary hypertension, or congenital heart disease. In all of these, the ECG appearance is the same.

The ECG changes associated with right ventricular hypertrophy are:

1. Right axis deviation
2. A dominant R wave (i.e. the R wave height is greater than the S wave depth) in V_1
3. 'Clockwise rotation' of the heart: as the right ventricle occupies more of the anterior surface of the chest and the septum is displaced laterally, the transition of the QRS complex in the chest leads from a right to a left ventricular configuration occurs in V_4–V_5 instead of in V_2–V_3. There is thus a persistent S wave in lead V_6, which normally does not show an S wave at all.
4. Inversion of the T wave in leads that 'look at' the right ventricle: V_1 and V_2, and occasionally V_3.

In extreme cases it is easy to diagnose right ventricular hypertrophy from the ECG. The next record came from a patient incapacitated with breathlessness due to thromboembolic pulmonary hypertension.

SEVERE RIGHT VENTRICULAR HYPERTROPHY

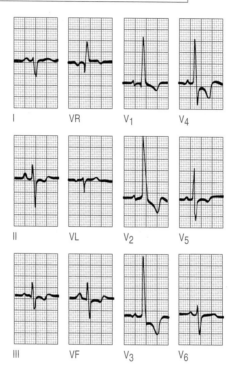

Note: Sinus rhythm with right axis deviation
Peaked P waves (especially in V_1) suggest right atrial hypertrophy
Dominant and very tall R waves in V_1–V_4
Deep S wave in V_6
Inverted T waves in V_1–V_5.

However, as in the case of the ECG in left ventricular hypertrophy, none of the ECG changes of right ventricular hypertrophy individually provide unequivocal evidence of right ventricular hypertrophy (Table 4.2). Conversely, it is possible to have marked right ventricular hypertrophy without all the ECG features being present.

Table 4.2 Causes of the ECG appearance of right ventricular hypertrophy

Right axis deviation	Normal in tall thin people
Dominant R wave in V_1	Normal variant Posterior infarction Wolff-Parkinson-White syndrome Right bundle branch block of any cause
Inverted T waves in V_1–V_3	Normal variant, especially in black people Anterior non-Q wave infarction Wolff-Parkinson-White syndrome Right bundle branch block of any cause Cardiomyopathy
Apparent clockwise rotation	Dextrocardia

Minor degrees of right axis deviation are seen in normal people, and a dominant R wave in V_1 is occasionally seen in normal people although it is never more than 3 or 4 mm tall. A dominant R wave in V_1 may also indicate a 'true posterior' myocardial infarction (see Ch. 3). There is a marked variation in T wave inversion in V_1 and V_2 in normal subjects (Ch. 1) and, particularly in Black people, the T wave can be inverted in V_2 and V_3.

The next ECG was recorded from a young woman who claimed to be dizzy and breathless, and who might have had pulmonary hypertension. In fact, her heart and lungs were entirely normal.

NORMAL ECG

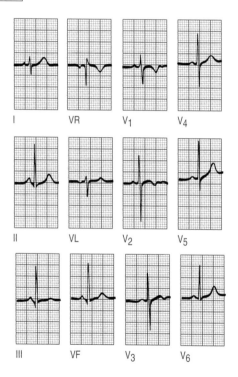

Note: Sinus rhythm with right axis deviation

T wave inversion in V_1–V_2

No other suggestion of right ventricular hypertrophy.

When the T wave inversion is more pronounced, the ECG might be confused with a non-Q wave infarction.

The next record was from a young woman who did have thromboembolic pulmonary hypertension, and who was quite breathless.

RIGHT VENTRICULAR HYPERTROPHY

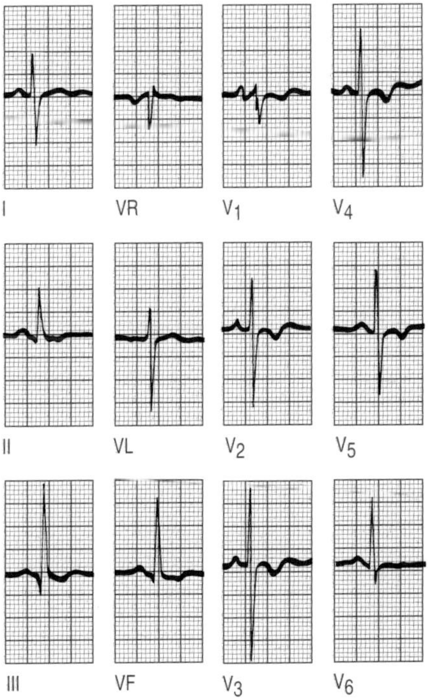

Note: Sinus rhythm

Dominant S wave in I shows right axis deviation, and this gives a clue to the cause of the T wave inversion

T wave inversion in V_1–V_5

In this case, there is no dominant R wave in V_1.

When anterior T wave inversion is associated with both right axis deviation and a dominant R wave in V_1, the diagnosis becomes much more obvious, and particularly so when the T wave inversion is most marked in V_1 and becomes progressively less marked in V_2 onwards.

RIGHT VENTRICULAR HYPERTROPHY

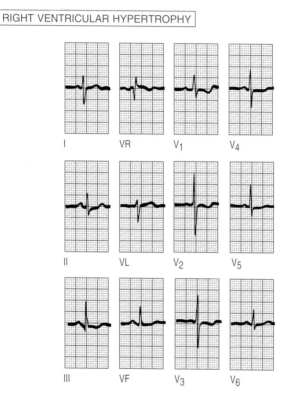

Note: Sinus rhythm
Right axis deviation
Dominant R wave in V_1
T wave inversion in V_1–V_4.

Marked 'clockwise rotation' can be a prominent feature of right ventricular hypertrophy.

RIGHT VENTRICULAR HYPERTROPHY

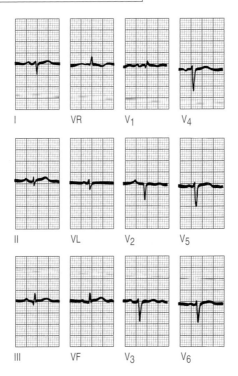

I	VR	V_1	V_4
II	VL	V_2	V_5
III	VF	V_3	V_6

Note: Sinus rhythm with right axis deviation
Small dominant R wave in V_1
Marked 'clockwise rotation' of the heart, with the right ventricle occupying the whole of the anterior surface of the heart. Even V_6 does not overlie the septum. All the chest leads show a right ventricular complex.

A deep S wave in V_6, without other ECG evidence of right ventricular hypertrophy, is characteristic of the ECGs of patients with chronic chest disease, such as obstructive airways disease.

CHRONIC LUNG DISEASE

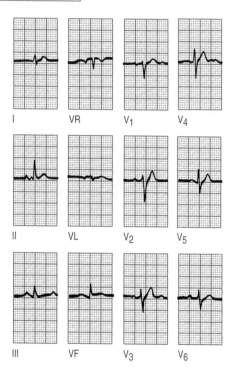

Note: The transition of the QRS complex from a right ventricular to a left ventricular type occurs in V_5, and there is a dominant S wave in V_6. There is no other evidence of right ventricular hypertrophy.

As in the case of the ECG in left ventricular hypertrophy, it is the appearance of changes in serial recordings that provides the best evidence of minor or moderate degrees of right ventricular hypertrophy.

In the majority of cases in which the ECG provides evidence of right ventricular hypertrophy, it is not possible to diagnose the underlying disease process. The exception to this is mitral stenosis, in which the obstruction of the flow of blood from the left atrium to the left ventricle causes left atrial hypertrophy – provided the heart is in sinus rhythm, this causes broad and bifid P waves. At the same time, raised pressure in the pulmonary veins causes pulmonary hypertension, and this in turn leads to right ventricular hypertrophy.

LA AND RV HYPERTROPHY IN MITRAL STENOSIS

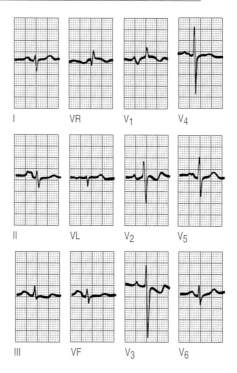

Note: Sinus rhythm, with broad and bifid P waves due to left atrial hypertrophy (especially in lead II)

Right axis deviation, a dominant R wave in V_1, inverted T waves in V_1–V_3, and an S wave in V_6 indicate right ventricular hypertrophy.

THE ECG IN CONGENITAL HEART DISEASE

The ECG provides a limited amount of help in the diagnosis of congenital heart disease by showing which chambers of the heart are enlarged. It is important to remember (see Ch. 1) that at birth, the ECG of a normal infant shows a pattern of 'right ventricular hypertrophy' and this gradually disappears during the first 2 years of life.

If the infant pattern persists beyond the age of 2 years, right ventricular hypertrophy is indeed present. If there is a left ventricular, or normal adult, pattern before this age, then left ventricular hypertrophy is probably present. In older children the same criteria for left and right ventricular hypertrophy apply as in adults.

Table 4.3 lists the common congenital disorders and the associated ECG appearance.

Table 4.3 ECG appearance in the common congenital disorders

ECG appearance	Congenital disorder
Right ventricular hypertrophy	Pulmonary hypertension of any cause, e.g. Eisenmenger's syndrome Severe pulmonary stenosis Fallot's tetralogy Transposition of the great arteries
Left ventricular hypertrophy	Aortic stenosis Coarctation of the aorta Mitral regurgitation Obstructive cardiomyopathy
Biventricular hypertrophy	Ventricular septal defect
Right atrial hypertrophy	Tricuspid stenosis
Right bundle branch block	Atrial septal defect Complex defects
Left axis deviation	Endocardial cushion defects Corrected transposition

RA AND RV HYPERTROPHY IN FALLOT'S TETRALOGY

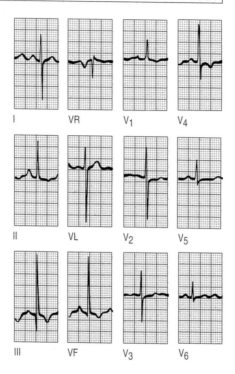

I   VR   V₁   V₄

II   VL   V₂   V₅

III   VF   V₃   V₆

Note: Peaked P wave in II indicates right atrial hypertrophy

Right axis deviation

Dominant R wave in V₁

This trace shows an 'S$_I$, Q$_{III}$, T$_{III}$' pattern, which shows that this combination of patterns is not diagnostic of pulmonary embolism.

WHAT TO DO

In most patients with breathlessness, the ECG does not contribute very much to diagnosis and management and the important thing is to treat the patient and not the ECG.

The ECG cannot diagnose heart failure, although by demonstrating ischaemia or enlargement of one or more of the cardiac chambers, it may help to elucidate the underlying disease that requires treatment. However, the symptoms of acute heart failure need empirical treatment whatever the ECG shows, and this should not be delayed while an ECG is being recorded.

Similarly, while the ECG can provide confirmatory evidence that breathlessness is due to a pulmonary embolus or chronic lung disease (Ch. 3), it is an unreliable way of making this diagnosis and treatment cannot depend on the ECG.

The ECG will not help in the diagnosis of anaemia, though it may show ischaemic changes.

In general, then, the management of the breathless patient does not depend on the ECG, but there are two important exceptions.

First, if breathlessness is due to heart failure which is secondary to an arrhythmia, then the ECG is essential both for diagnosis and for monitoring the response to therapy.

Second, the ECG has an important role in the timing of surgery for valve disease, particularly aortic valve disease. In aortic stenosis, left ventricular enlargement may not be obvious on examination even when the valve lesion is severe. Even in an asymptomatic patient, evidence of left ventricular hypertrophy on the ECG is an indication for urgent echocardiography and cardiac catheterization with a view to surgery, because when aortic stenosis is sufficiently severe to cause such changes the prognosis is poor. Serial recording of the ECG is one investigation that can be useful when monitoring the progress of patients with mitral and aortic valve disease, because the appearance of any changes will at least be a relative indication for surgery.

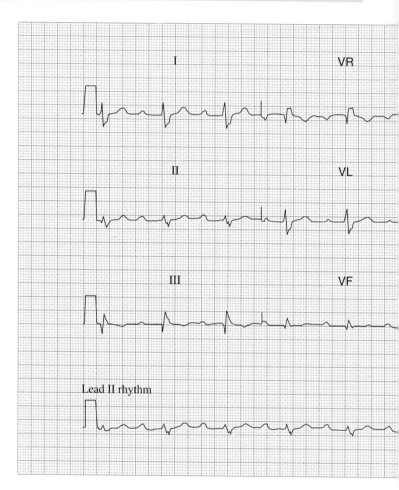

This ECG was recorded from a 60-year-old man suffering from congestive cardiac failure. He had never had chest pain. His heart was enlarged, his jugular venous pressure was elevated, and at the cardiac apex a pansystolic murmur and a third sound were audible. The ECG shows:

- Sinus rhythm
- First degree block
- Right axis deviation

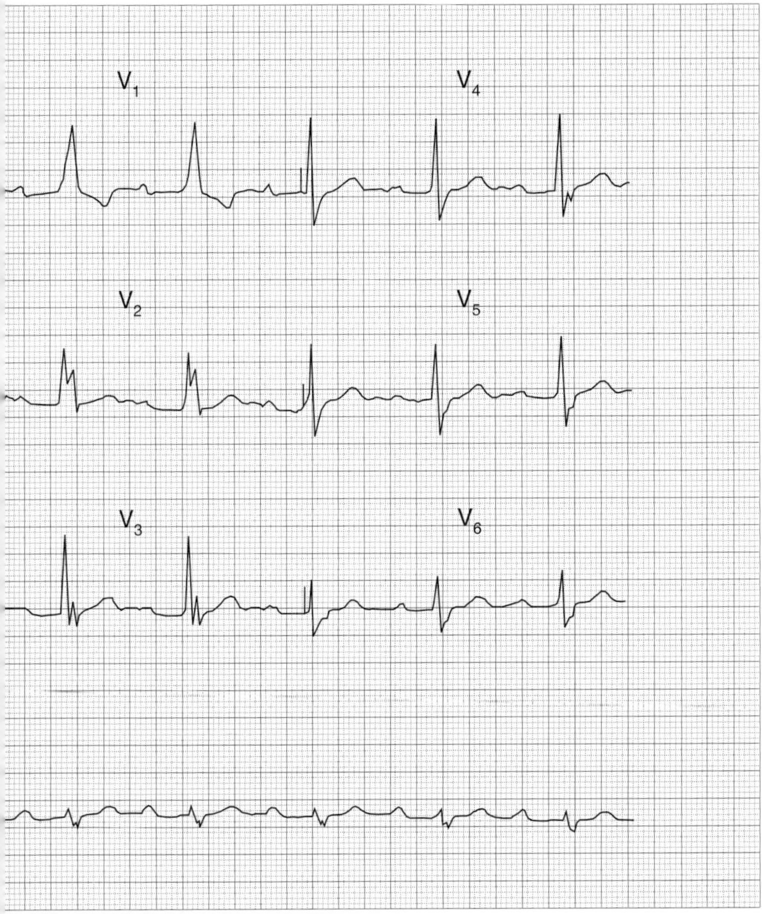

- Broad QRS complexes, with a dominant R wave in V_1 and a slight notch on the upstroke – the RSR^1 pattern is better seen in V_2
- Deep and slurred S wave in V_6.

Interpretation:

Right bundle branch block. First degree block indicates a further conduction abnormality, which could be in the AV node, the His bundle, or the left bundle branch.

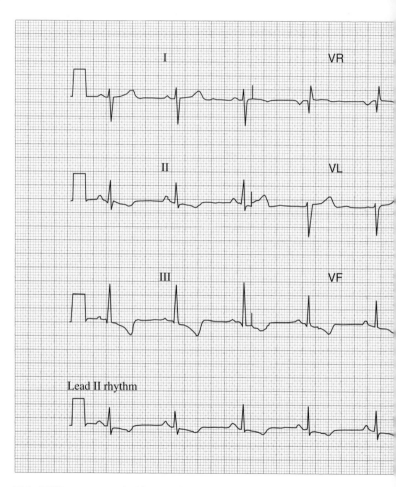

This ECG was recorded from a 55-year-old woman who had been increasingly short of breath since she had had a hysterectomy 6 months previously. She had not had any chest pain.
The ECG shows:
- Sinus rhythm
- Normal conduction intervals
- Right axis deviation

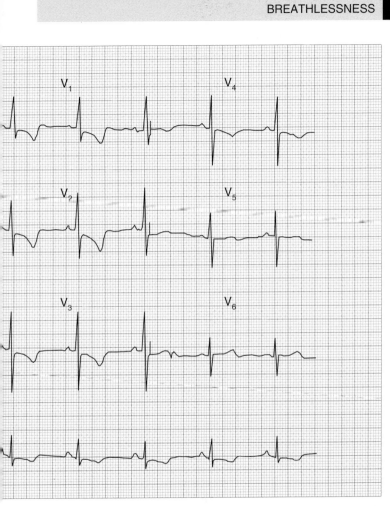

- Dominant R wave in lead V_1 and dominant S wave in lead V_6 ('clockwise rotation')
- Inverted T waves in III, VF, V_1–V_4.

Interpretation:

Right ventricular hypertrophy, suggesting that the breathlessness may be due to recurrent pulmonary emboli following the hysterectomy.

CHAPTER 5

The effect of non-cardiac disease on the ECG

The ECG is not a good method for investigating or diagnosing any condition that is not primarily cardiac. However, some generalized diseases affect the ECG and it is important to recognize this and not assume that a patient has heart disease simply because his or her ECG seems abnormal. In this context it is also essential to remember the wide range of ECG patterns seen in healthy subjects, and to recognize that technical artefacts in the ECG can sometimes suggest the presence of heart disease.

This chapter deals first with some of the common artefacts in the ECG and then with the effects on the ECG of hypothermia, thyroid disease, malignancy, electrolyte imbalance, digoxin and other drugs.

ARTEFACTS IN ECG RECORDINGS

Improper electrode placement

If the electrodes are wrongly attached to the limbs there will be abnormalities in the height of the P waves, QRS complexes, and T waves, and the cardiac axis may seem bizarre. The ECG will, however, be normal in the V leads. When the P wave is upside down in leads other than VR, despite the patient being in sinus rhythm with a normal PR interval, or when the cardiac axis is difficult to calculate, improper electrode attachment should be suspected and the recording repeated.

?NORMAL ECG

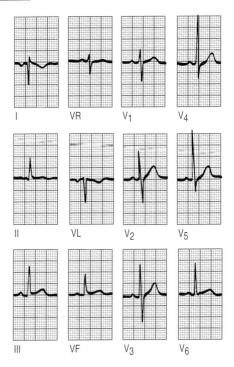

Note: In this ECG the right arm electrode has been attached to the left arm and vice versa. The P wave is upside down in I and VL. The appearance of the V leads is normal.

Dextrocardia causes abnormalities in the standard leads similar to those caused by improper electrode attachment, but the pattern of the chest leads is also abnormal. Leads that normally 'look at' the left ventricle (V_5 and V_6) record a 'right ventricular' complex (Ch. 1).

When an ECG appears odd it is always prudent to suspect a technical error and repeat the recording.

?NORMAL ECG

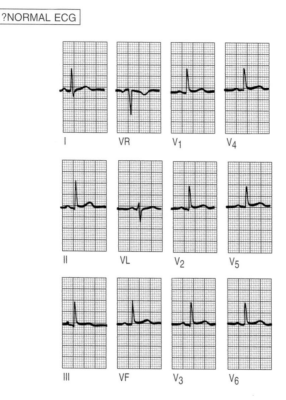

Note: This record was made with a single-channel ECG recorder. The ECG in the standard leads is normal. In all the 'chest leads' the QRS complex is identical, and is the same as in VF. The 'chest leads' have been recorded with the lead selector left in the VF position.

The effects of abnormal muscle movement

The contraction of any muscle is initiated by depolarization of the muscle cells, and although ECG recorders are designed to be especially sensitive to the frequencies of cardiac muscle, the ECG will record the contraction of skeletal muscle. The most common pattern of 'ECG abnormality' is a high-frequency oscillation due to general muscular tension in a patient who is not properly relaxed. This is accentuated when the patient is cold and shivering.

HYPOTHERMIA

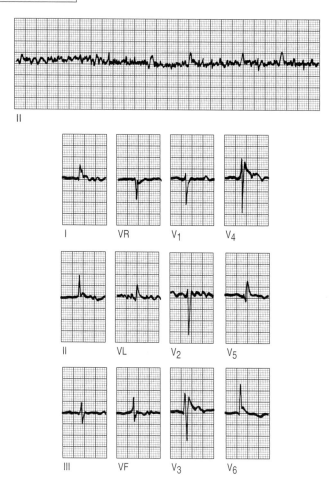

II

I

VR

V₁

V₄

II

VL

V₂

V₅

III

VF

V₃

V₆

Note: Coarse 'muscle tremor' obscures any P waves that might
be present, but the irregularity of the QRS complexes in
the top (rhythm) strip suggests that the rhythm is atrial
fibrillation. The rhythm strip was recorded while the patient
was shivering severely.

The ECG of a hypothermic patient may show, in addition to the effects of generalized tremor, a hump (a J wave) at the end of the QRS complex. It is difficult to distinguish these in the preceding record. The J waves are clearly seen in the next record, which came from a hypothermic patient who was not shivering.

HYPOTHERMIA

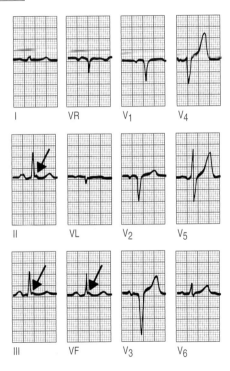

Note: The ECG is normal apart from J waves at the end of the QRS complexes. These are most clearly seen in II, III and VF (arrowed).

Sustained involuntary tremors cause rhythmic ECG abnormalities that may be confused with cardiac arrhythmias.

PARKINSONISM

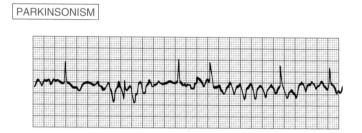

Note: Muscle tremor at 5 per second gives an appearance resembling atrial flutter. The irregular QRS complexes may indicate that the rhythm is atrial fibrillation. This record demonstrates the importance of looking at the patient as well as at the ECG.

THE ECG IN SYSTEMIC DISEASES

Cardiac involvement in a generalized disorder, particularly one that causes infiltration or the abnormal deposition of substances in the myocardium, causes arrhythmias and conduction defects.

Thyroid disease

Thyrotoxicosis is probably the most common disorder that may present as a cardiac problem. Particularly in old age, it may cause atrial fibrillation, usually with a rapid ventricular response which is difficult to control with digoxin. An elderly patient may complain mainly of palpitations or of the symptoms of heart failure, and arterial embolization may occur. The usual symptoms of thyrotoxicosis may be mild or even absent.

THYROTOXICOSIS

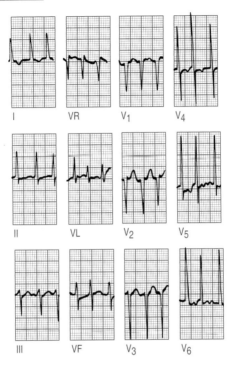

I   VR   V₁   V₄

II   VL   V₂   V₅

III   VF   V₃   V₆

Note: Atrial fibrillation with a ventricular rate of about 200 per minute
The T waves are inverted in the anterior and lateral leads, indicating probable ischaemia.

In myxoedema there will usually be a sinus bradycardia and sometimes non-specific ST segment/T wave changes. If there is a pericardial effusion, the QRS complexes may be small.

Malignancy

Malignant disease with secondary deposits in the heart can cause atrial fibrillation, and a deposit placed appropriately in the conducting system can cause complete heart block. In Western countries, malignancy is the commonest cause of large pericardial effusions (tuberculosis being more common in underdeveloped countries). The combination of an arrhythmia with small complexes suggests mediastinal malignancy.

MALIGNANT PERICARDIAL EFFUSION

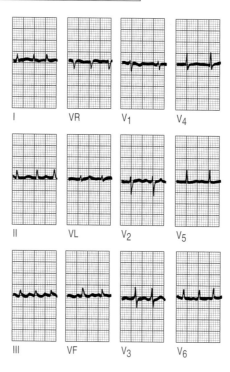

Note: Atrial fibrillation, with a ventricular rate of about 150 per minute
Small QRS complexes suggest the presence of a pericardial effusion.

Electrolyte imbalance

Hypokalaemia and hypocalcaemia

Hypokalaemia occurs most commonly as the result of diuretic therapy. It prolongs the QT interval, which is measured from the onset of the QRS complex to the end of the T wave. In hypokalaemia, the T wave is flattened and is followed by a further low-amplitude deflection called a U wave. U waves are commonly seen in normal records, particularly in the anterior chest leads, V_2–V_4, but in a normal ECG the T wave is not flattened (see Ch. 1). The next ECG was recorded from a patient with a serum potassium level of 1.9 mmol/l.

HYPOKALAEMIA

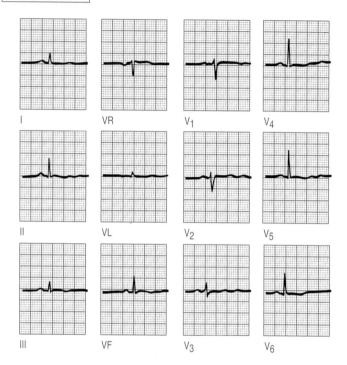

I VR V₁ V₄

II VL V₂ V₅

III VF V₃ V₆

Note: Sinus rhythm with normal QRS complexes
In all leads the T waves are flattened. It
is difficult to measure the QT interval, but it
is probably 440 ms
U waves are present in most leads.

Hypokalaemia can also cause ST segment depression and first
or second degree heart block.
The QT interval is also prolonged in hypocalcaemia, and in
severe rheumatic carditis.

Hyperkalaemia and hypercalcaemia

Hyperkalaemia causes flattening of the P waves, widening of the QRS complexes, symmetrical peaking of the T waves and loss of the ST segment. Fatal arrhythmias may occur.

Hypercalcaemia shortens the QT interval.

The next ECG came from a patient with a serum potassium level of 5.9 mmol/l.

HYPERKALAEMIA

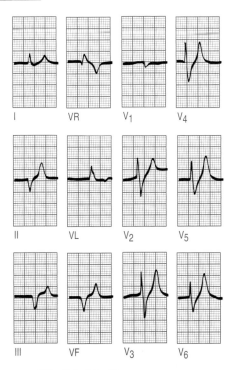

Note: P waves difficult to identify
Sinus rhythm with left axis deviation
T waves are peaked in all leads
ST segment not clearly defined.

Magnesium imbalance

The effects of high or low serum magnesium levels are similar to those of high and low potassium.

Summary

Table 5.1 summarizes the effects of electrolyte abnormalities.

Table 5.1 The effects of electrolyte imbalance on the ECG

| | Serum electrolyte level | |
	Low	High
Potassium or magnesium	Flat T waves Prominent U waves Depressed ST segment First or second degree block	Flat P waves Widening of QRS complexes (nonspecific intraventricular conduction delay) Tall peaked T waves Disappearance of ST segment
Calcium	Prolonged QT interval (due to long ST segment)	Short QT interval, with loss of ST segment

THE EFFECTS OF MEDICATION ON THE ECG

Digitalis

The main use of digoxin and the other drugs related to digitalis is to block atrioventricular conduction and so to slow the ventricular rate in atrial fibrillation. Provided AV conduction is normal, atrial fibrillation will usually be associated with a rapid ventricular response. A slow ventricular rate, particularly with regular QRS complexes, suggests digitalis effect. Digitalis also causes downsloping depression of the ST segments with inversion of the T waves, and these changes are most pronounced in the left lateral leads (VL, V_5–V_6). Digitalis tends to shorten the QT interval.

DIGITALIS EFFECT

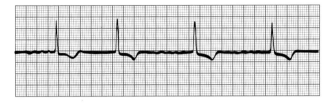

Note: Atrial fibrillation, with a ventricular rate of about 50 per minute
The ST segments slope downwards and the T waves are inverted, giving a 'reverse tick' appearance.

The effects of digoxin on the ECG must be differentiated from those of ischaemia, which causes horizontal ST segment depression. Both changes can sometimes be recognized in a single ECG record.

ISCHAEMIA AND DIGOXIN

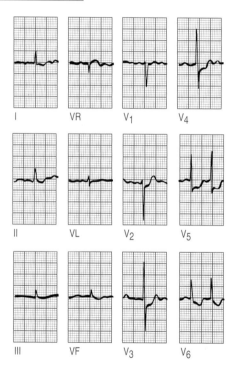

Note: Atrial fibrillation, with a ventricular rate of 150 per minute at times

In V_3–V_5 there is horizontal ST segment depression, suggesting ischaemia

In V_6 the ST segments slope downwards and the T waves are inverted; these changes are probably due to digoxin.

Digoxin toxicity can cause almost any cardiac arrhythmia, including bradycardias and tachycardias. The most classical digoxin-induced arrhythmias are atrioventricular block, atrial tachycardia with block, multifocal ventricular extrasystoles, and sometimes ventricular tachycardia. These arrhythmias are particularly likely to occur in the presence of hypokalaemia.

DIGOXIN TOXICITY

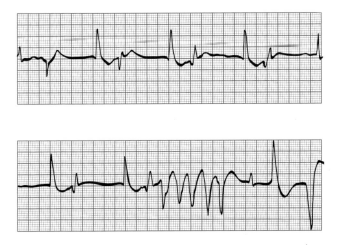

Note: The two strips form a continuous record. The basic rhythm is atrial fibrillation, and the upright QRS complexes are probably the normally conducted beats. Each of these is followed by a predominantly downward QRS complex, which represents a ventricular extrasystole. In the lower strip there is a short run of ventricular tachycardia.

Anti-arrhythmic drugs

All the anti-arrhythmic drugs of the 'class I' type (quinidine, lignocaine, disopyramide, flecainide etc.) can actually cause arrhythmias. Some prolong the QT interval (and amiodarone can also have this effect), but others do not. All cause ventricular tachycardia, which is usually of the 'torsades de pointes' type, in which the QRS complexes change progressively due to changing re-entry pathways (Ch. 6).

QUINIDINE TOXICITY

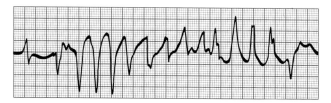

Note: A single sinus beat is followed by a run of ventricular tachycardia. The QRS complexes initially point downwards, but then change progressively to an upright configuration. This writhing appearance is referred to as the torsades de pointes variety of ventricular tachycardia.

Other drugs

Tricyclic antidepressants cause arrhythmias, and lithium causes sinus node slowing and T wave abnormalities.

WHAT TO DO

The ECG is not a reliable aid in the diagnosis of problems in which the heart is affected only as part of an overall disease process. In most cases, for example in malignant disease, non-cardiac symptoms and signs will predominate, but in others (particularly thyrotoxicosis in the elderly) a cardiac abnormality may be the primary feature of the illness.

As always in medicine, the first thing to remember is not to place undue reliance on a single investigation, and the second is not to be satisfied with the immediate diagnosis. If the ECG reveals atrial fibrillation, think about its cause. If the ECG raises the possibility of a pericardial effusion, ask whether this is consistent with the patient's appearance and then think what the causes of a pericardial effusion could be. An ECG will define the nature of a conduction defect or an arrhythmia but will not indicate its cause, and the cause of the arrhythmia is the prime diagnosis. Always consider the possibility that an ECG abnormality may be related to medical therapy, and remember that the patient's history and physical signs will always be more important than the ECG itself.

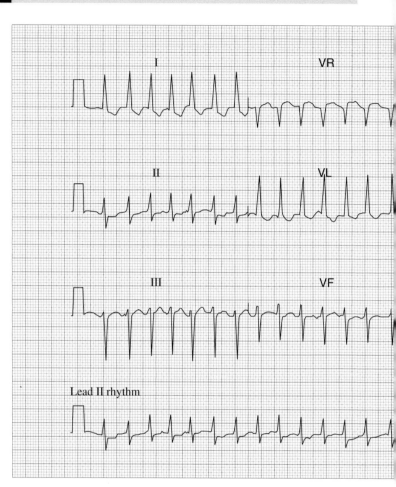

This ECG was recorded from a 75-year-old woman who had suddenly developed palpitations and breathlessness 1 month previously. Despite treatment, her symptoms had not improved. The ECG shows:

- Atrial fibrillation, with a ventricular rate varying between 100–200 per minute
- Loss of R wave in V_3, with a normal R wave in V_4
- Downsloping ST segments and inverted T waves in the lateral leads.

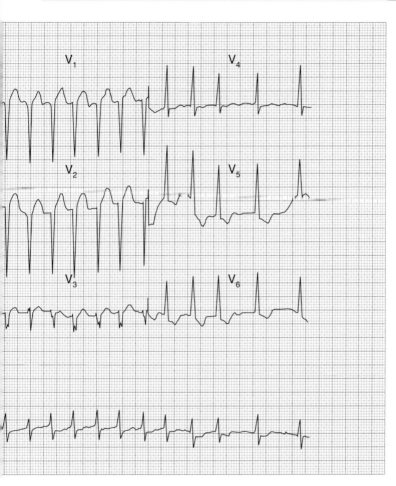

Interpretation:

Atrial fibrillation with an uncontrolled ventricular rate. The lack of an R wave in V_3 could indicate an old anterior infarction. The ST segment/T wave changes suggest that she is being treated with digoxin. An old lady who develops atrial fibrillation, particularly when it is not controlled by digoxin, may be thyrotoxic.

CHAPTER 6

The physiological basis of the ECG

It is perfectly possible, and not unreasonable, to look at the ECG simply as a tool with which to investigate patients who have symptoms or signs suggesting cardiovascular disease. The ECG can be used in this way with little understanding of the physiological processes involved. However, it is easier to work out the cause of many ECG abnormalities by thinking in physiological terms, and several ECG abnormalities that are unimportant in that they do not cause symptoms or any impairment of cardiac function are both interesting and important in demonstrating how the heart works.

THE CELLULAR BASIS OF THE ECG

Contraction of a muscle cell is initiated by an electrical change called depolarization. When an individual muscle cell is at rest, its surface is positively charged and its interior is negatively charged; the potential difference across the cell membrane is about −90 mV. An electrical stimulus can cause a sudden, rapid influx of sodium ions (positively charged) from the extracellular fluid into the cell, so causing the inside of the cell to become positively charged compared with the outside: the transmembrane potential briefly rises to about +30 mV. This change in the transmembrane potential is called depolarization.

TRANSMEMBRANE POTENTIAL AND IONIC FLUX ACROSS A
MYOCARDIAL CELL MEMBRANE

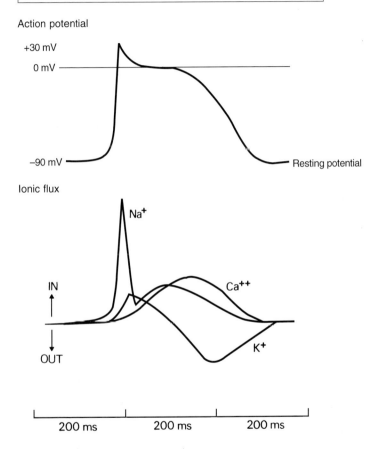

The initial influx of sodium rapidly ceases, and there is an early
and partial repolarization to a membrane potential of about zero.
Then follows a slow entry of more sodium ions and also of calcium
ions (also positively charged) into the muscle cell. The entry of
these ions together would tend to cause the transmembrane

potential to rise again, but the influx of sodium and calcium ions is balanced by an outflow of potassium ions. The net electrical result of these later ionic fluxes is that the transmembrane potential of the muscle cell is held constant at about zero for some 200 ms. Thereafter, calcium and sodium ions move out of the cell and 'repolarization' occurs, with a fall of the transmembrane potential to the resting level of −90 mV. Together, these transmembrane potential changes, depolarization and repolarization constitute the 'action potential'.

When the surface charge of a myocardial cell changes polarity from positive to negative, there will be a movement of positive ions in the extracellular fluid away from the adjacent 'resting' cell towards the depolarized cell. This movement of positive ions away from the resting cells triggers depolarization in them, and depolarization therefore spreads from one myocardial cell to another. Depolarization therefore spreads outwards, like an advancing wave in all directions, from the cell that was first depolarized.

THE SHAPE OF THE ECG

It may be difficult to grasp the relationship between the action potential of an individual myocyte, the wave of depolarization caused by the spread of action potentials through the heart, and the ECG that is recorded from the surface of the body. The important thing to remember is that the ECG represents an average: an average of all the action potentials at any one time, and an average direction of the depolarization wave over time. Because each ECG complex (P wave, QRS complex and T wave) represents an average of the electrical activity of all the myocardial cells over the time taken for the depolarization and repolarization of the whole myocardium, it is meaningless to try to superimpose P waves, QRS complexes and T waves on the diagram on page 239.

Each ECG lead (that is, each of the six standard or limb leads, and the six chest leads) compares the potential difference between two electrodes. This is easiest to understand if we think of one of the chest leads, such as V_6. V_6 measures the potential difference between an electrode attached to the chest and an 'indifferent' electrode (made of a combination of the electrodes attached to the arms and the left leg, the right leg electrode being connected to earth). The position of lead V_6 is defined arbitrarily, but in most people it roughly corresponds to the cardiac apex.

When all the myocardial cells are depolarized there is no potential difference between the V_6 electrode and the indifferent electrode, and the ECG forms its baseline. As the heart – and for this purpose let us just consider the ventricles – is depolarized, the indifferent electrode records a steadily increasing state of depolarization. This would be recorded in exactly the same way by V_6 except for a crucial fact: V_6 is more influenced by events occurring nearer to it – so as the depolarization wave moves towards V_6, the potential difference between the V_6 electrode and the indifferent electrode increases. The ECG recorder is arranged so that a depolarization wave moving towards an electrode causes an upward deflection – hence the development of the R wave in V_6. When all the cells in the ventricles are depolarized, there is once again no potential difference between the V_6 electrode and the indifferent electrode – the ECG returns to baseline, forming the ST segment.

Repolarization involves the opposite movement of ions compared with depolarization, so one might have expected the effects of repolarization on the ECG (the T wave) to be in the opposite direction compared with those of depolarization (the QRS complex). However, repolarization occurs in the opposite direction anatomically from depolarization because of differences in the properties of myocardial cells in different parts of the heart. Whereas the average depolarization wave spreads roughly from the base of the heart towards the apex, repolarization begins in the cells depolarized last (at the apex) and the repolarization wave moves away from the apex towards the base. This has the effect of inverting the repolarization wave – that is, making the T wave upright rather than inverted.

All the same principles apply to the P wave, which represents atrial depolarization. In theory there should be a repolarization wave for the atria corresponding to the T wave caused by repolarization of the ventricles, but in practice atrial repolarization is never seen on the ECG, because it is too diffuse and too prolonged.

CONDUCTION OF THE DEPOLARIZATION WAVE

Depolarization is normally initiated in the sinoatrial (SA) node, and the depolarization wave is conducted through the atrial muscle to the atrioventricular (AV) node. In the AV node conduction is markedly slowed, but from this node originates the tract of specialized myocytes which constitutes the only normal connection between the atria and ventricles, and which is called the bundle of His. The bundle of His passes from the atria to the ventricles close to the upper part of the tricuspid valve, and in the interventricular septum divides into left and right bundle branches. The left branch divides again, into antero-superior and postero-inferior branches. Thus three main divisions, or fascicles, of the bundle of His conduct the depolarization wave rapidly to the branching network of conducting fibres called the Purkinje tissue. The depolarization wave thus finally arrives at the ventricular myocardial cells.

This spread of depolarization is called conduction, and all cardiac muscle cells can conduct a depolarization wave. As described above, conduction can occur directly from one muscle cell to another because depolarization is triggered when ions move away from resting cells towards depolarized cells, but this is a relatively slow process compared to conduction in specialized conduction tissues. The conduction velocity from one atrial muscle cell to another is about 1.0 metre per second (m/s), compared with 0.2 m/s in the AV node, 4.0 m/s in the His bundle and Purkinje tissue, and 0.5 m/s in the ventricular muscle.

CONDUCTION AND THE ELECTROCARDIOGRAM

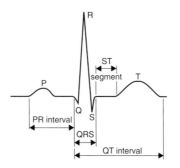

The P wave is normally small and broad because the combined muscle mass of the atria is considerably less than that of the ventricles and conduction through the atria is slow. The segment of the ECG between the end of the P wave and the beginning of the QRS complex has little clinical importance, but will be at the ECG baseline because it represents the time when the atria are fully depolarized. The PR interval represents the time taken for depolarization to spread from the SA node through the atria and the AV node to the interventricular septum, which is the first part of the ventricular muscle to depolarize. Provided the conduction of depolarization through the ventricular muscle mass is normal, depolarization of both ventricles is completed in 120 ms, and so three small squares of ECG paper is the upper limit for the width of the normal QRS complex.

When ventricular depolarization is complete, the ECG normally returns to its baseline, forming the ST segment (but the ST segment is displaced upward in infarction, and downward in ischaemia and during treatment with digoxin or quinidine). The length of the ST segment corresponds very crudely to the period between the early and late depolarization of the ventricular myocytes, but this is difficult to measure and is of no clinical importance.

The T wave represents repolarization of the ventricles, and the height and direction of the T wave are affected by many things, including ischaemia, infarction, and electrolyte imbalance. The length of the T wave is difficult to measure and varies considerably from lead to lead, so the QT interval is usually taken as the best indication of the time taken for repolarization of the ventricles.

CONDUCTION DEFECTS

The conduction of depolarization can be delayed or 'blocked' anywhere along the pathway from the SA node to the ventricular muscle, and the sites of conduction defects can usually be deduced from the surface ECG.

POSSIBLE SITES FOR CONDUCTION BLOCK

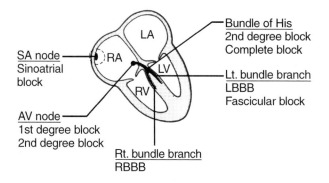

Sinoatrial block

In sinoatrial block, the SA node depolarizes normally but the depolarization wave fails to penetrate the atrium.

SINOATRIAL BLOCK

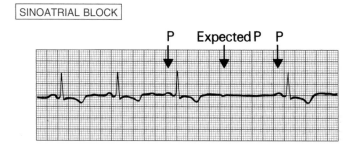

Note: Sinus rhythm for three beats, then a 'sinus pause'. The expected P wave is not seen, but the SA node must have been depolarized because the next P wave appears at the predicted time.

Intra-atrial conduction delay

Depolarization spreads throughout the atrial muscle, so conduction defects do not occur, but activation of the whole of the atrial myocardium may take longer than normal if the left atrium is hypertrophied. This causes the broad bifid P wave seen in the ECGs of patients with mitral stenosis, as long as they remain in sinus rhythm (Ch. 4).

AV node and His bundle block

The PR interval (the period from the onset of the P wave to the first deflection of the QRS complex) measures the time taken for the depolarization wave to spread from the SA node, through the atria and the AV node, and down the His bundle to the interventricular septum. If the PR interval is prolonged, or if the P wave is not followed by a QRS complex, a conduction defect must be present either in the AV node itself or in the His bundle. It is not possible to tell from the surface ECG which of these two sites is involved.

   The passage of the depolarization wave down the His bundle can be detected if an electrode is placed close to the His bundle: this can be done by passing an electrode catheter up a femoral vein and positioning it just through the tricuspid valve. The electrical activity associated with atrial depolarization recorded in this way is called an 'A' wave rather than a 'P' wave, and that associated with ventricular depolarization is called a 'V' wave rather than a 'QRS' complex. Depolarization of the His bundle itself is shown as a sharp deflection called the 'H spike'.

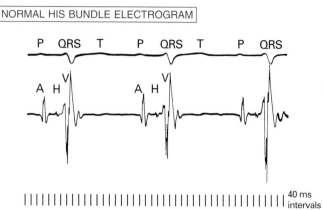

NORMAL HIS BUNDLE ELECTROGRAM

P QRS T   P QRS T   P QRS

A H V   A H V

|||||||||||||||||||||||||||||||||||||||||||||||| 40 ms intervals

Note: Upper trace shows the usual ECG recorded from the body surface. The P waves, QRS complexes and T waves are broad and flat because the record was made with a fast paper speed.

The lower trace shows the intracardiac recording. The 'A' and 'V' waves correspond to the P waves and QRS complexes, but have a totally different appearance.

His bundle depolarization is shown as a small spike labelled 'H'.

The AH interval thus measures the time taken for the depolarization wave to spread from the SA node to the His bundle. Most of this period is due to delay within the AV node. In normal subjects the AH interval is between 55 and 120 ms. The HV interval (normal range 35–55 ms) measures the time taken for depolarization to spread from the His bundle to the first part of the interventricular septum.

First degree block

When each atrial depolarization is followed by ventricular depolarization but atrioventricular conduction is slow, the PR interval on the surface ECG is prolonged and 'first degree block' is said to be present. This may indicate many varieties of heart disease (for example, it is seen in acute myocardial infarction and acute rheumatic carditis) but in itself it does not impair cardiac function, and does not cause symptoms.

| 1st DEGREE BLOCK |

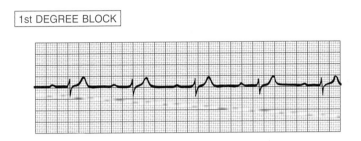

Note: Sinus rhythm
PR interval is constant at 360 ms.

First degree block commonly occurs in the AV node. A His bundle electrogram therefore records a prolonged AH interval but a normal HV interval, because conduction in the distal part of the His bundle is normal.

| HIS ELECTROGRAM: 1st DEGREE BLOCK |

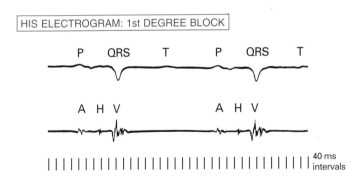

Note: Upper record shows surface ECG
Lower record shows His electrogram: AH interval is prolonged at 150 ms, but the HV interval is normal at 70 ms.

Second degree block

When atrial depolarization intermittently fails to induce ventricular depolarization, 'second degree block' exists, and this can result from conduction failure anywhere in the AV node or His bundle. There are three varieties:

(a) When most beats are conducted normally but occasionally a P wave is not followed by a QRS complex, second degree block of the 'Mobitz Type 2' variety is said to be present. The conduction defect is thought to be below the AV node, in the bundle of His. This does not in itself cause symptoms, and its only importance is that it may precede the development of complete block.

2nd DEGREE BLOCK (MOBITZ TYPE 2)

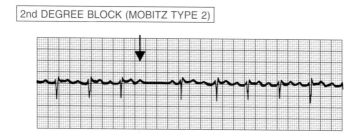

Note: Sinus rhythm with a normal PR interval
One P wave (arrowed) is not followed by a QRS complex.

(b) When the PR interval lengthens progressively with each beat and then a P wave is not conducted and is not followed by a QRS complex, the 'Wenckebach phenomenon' is present. The conduction abnormality in this case is within the AV node.

2nd DEGREE BLOCK (WENCKEBACH)

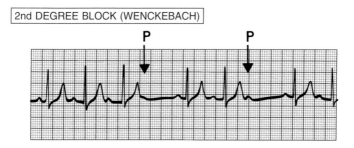

Note: Three beats with progressively longer PR intervals are
followed by a non-conducted P wave (arrowed). The next
PR interval is short, but this is followed by a longer PR
interval and then another non-conducted beat.

(c) When alternate P waves are not conducted, second degree
block of the '2:1' type is said to be present.

2nd DEGREE BLOCK (2:1)

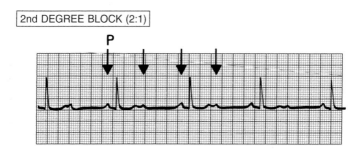

Note: The conducted beats have a normal PR interval, but
alternate P waves are not followed by a QRS complex.

A His bundle electrogram demonstrates the site of second degree block. In the case of 2:1 block this will usually be in the His bundle rather than the AV node – so a normal H (or His) spike will be seen, but in the non-conducted beats the H spike will not be followed by a V wave.

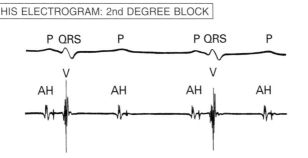

HIS ELECTROGRAM: 2nd DEGREE BLOCK

Note: Upper trace shows the surface ECG; as in the case of the other His electrograms the paper speed is fast, so the P–QRS–T complexes are flattened and spread out.
Lower trace shows first a normal A wave, H spike and V wave, but then an A wave and an H spike with no V wave. The sequence is then repeated.

Second degree block of the Mobitz 2 and Wenckebach types does not cause symptoms, but 2:1 block may cause heart failure if the ventricular rate is slow enough.

Third degree block

Third degree, or complete, heart block results either from His bundle disease or from bilateral bundle branch block. A narrow QRS complex indicates that the rhythm originates within the His bundle itself below the block, but a wide QRS complex indicates that ventricular depolarization originates in the Purkinje system.

COMPLETE (3rd DEGREE) BLOCK

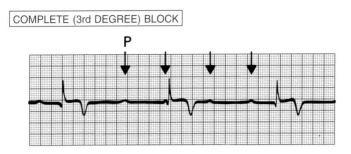

Note: No relationship between P waves (arrowed) and QRS complexes. The QRS complexes are normal, indicating that the origin of ventricular depolarization is within the His bundle. The ventricular rate is 30 per minute.

When complete heart block complicates an acute inferior infarction, the ventricular rate is usually about 50 per minute. The classical ventricular escape rate of 20–30 per minute is usually seen when complete block results from fibrosis of the His bundle.

COMPLETE (3rd DEGREE) BLOCK

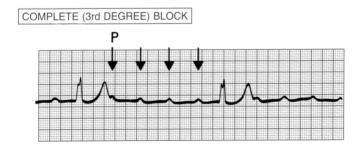

Note: No relationship between P waves (arrowed) and QRS complexes
Wide QRS complexes, with a ventricular rate of 22 per minute.

Complete heart block does impair cardiac performance: the effect of synchronized atrial and ventricular contraction is lost and, more importantly, cardiac output falls because of the slow heart rate.

Bundle branch block

When the His bundle conducts normally but one of the bundle branches is blocked, the PR interval is normal but the QRS complex is widened because of the late depolarization of the ventricle normally supplied by the bundle branch which is blocked. Bundle branch block does not significantly impair cardiac function, and in itself will not be responsible for any symptoms the patient may have.

Right bundle branch block is characterized by an RSR^1 pattern in V_1.

RIGHT BUNDLE BRANCH BLOCK

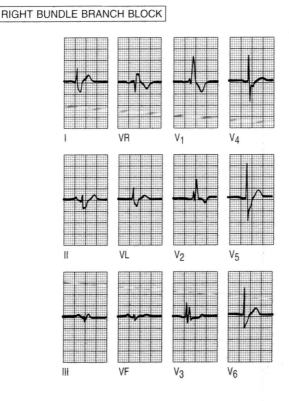

Note: Sinus rhythm with a normal PR interval

Right axis deviation

RSR^1 pattern in V_1; the dominant R wave is characteristic of RBBB, and does not indicate RV hypertrophy

Wide and slurred S wave in V_6.

Left bundle branch block is characterized by a loss of the septal Q wave and the notching of the QRS complex in the lateral leads.

LEFT BUNDLE BRANCH BLOCK

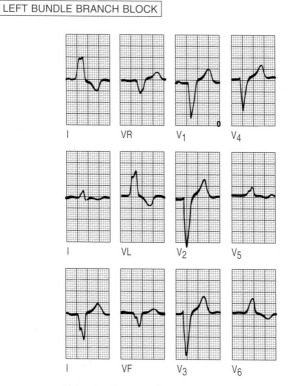

V leads at ½ sensitivity

Note: Sinus rhythm

Broad QRS complexes with notch in the R wave in I, III, VL, VF and V₅

Remember that inverted T waves are associated with bundle branch block, and have no other significance.

If a bundle branch block is associated with first degree block, it is likely that the remaining bundle branch is diseased and that bilateral bundle branch block (causing third degree block) is imminent.

1st DEGREE BLOCK AND BUNDLE BRANCH BLOCK

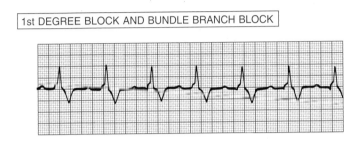

Note: Sinus rhythm

PR interval 280 ms (first degree block)

Broad QRS complexes and inverted T waves indicate bundle branch block, but in a single monitoring lead such as this it is not possible to say which bundle branch is blocked.

Fascicular block

The right bundle branch is a single structure, but the left bundle branch divides into two further branches or fascicles. Depolarization spreads into the left ventricle through these fascicles, and the average of these two directions of depolarization as seen from the front is called the frontal plane vector or cardiac axis.

THE NORMAL CARDIAC AXIS

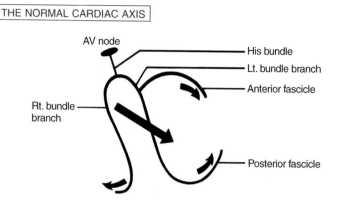

Note: Small arrows show the direction of spread of depolarization through the main branches of the His bundle. The broad arrow shows the average direction of spread of depolarization in these three branches as seen from the front. This is the 'cardiac axis'.

Failure of conduction in the antero-superior branch of the left bundle (left anterior fascicular block or 'left anterior hemiblock') means that the left ventricle has to be depolarized through the posterior fascicle. The average direction of depolarization, the cardiac axis, therefore swings upwards and causes left axis deviation.

LEFT ANTERIOR HEMIBLOCK

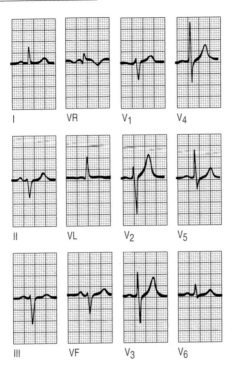

Note: Sinus rhythm with a normal PR interval
The average direction of depolarization in the standard leads is mainly towards I and VL, and away from both II and III, which show dominant S waves. This is left axis deviation.

Failure of conduction in the posterior inferior fascicle (left posterior hemiblock) causes the cardiac axis to swing to the right, and this is shown by a deep S wave in lead I. This is seen much less often than left anterior hemiblock. Left posterior hemiblock can be recognized by the association of right axis deviation and some evidence of left ventricular disease, without anything to suggest right ventricular hypertrophy.

Bifascicular block

A combination of right bundle branch block and left anterior hemiblock indicates disease of two of the three main ventricular conduction pathways. This is an example of 'bifascicular' block.

BIFASCICULAR BLOCK

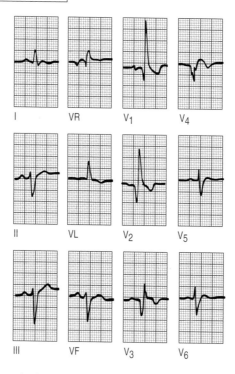

Note: Sinus rhythm with a normal PR interval
Left axis deviation
RSR[1] pattern in V_1 and deep S wave in V_6 indicate RBBB.

RHYTHMS RESULTING FROM CARDIAC AUTOMATICITY

Myocardial cells are only depolarized when they are stimulated, but the cells of the sinoatrial node, those around the atrioventricular node (the 'junctional' cells) and those of the conducting pathways all possess the property of spontaneous depolarization or 'automaticity'. The action potential wave-form of these cells is quite different from that of the myocardial cells: the transmembrane potential slowly becomes less negative during diastole and when it reaches a critical threshold, depolarization occurs. This should be contrasted with the 'triggered' depolarization of myocytes shown on page 239.

TRANSMEMBRANE POTENTIAL WITH AUTOMATICITY

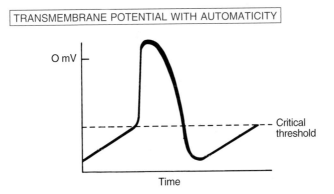

O mV

Critical
threshold

Time

Sinus arrhythmia

This automatic depolarization is quite regular, although it can be influenced by physiological and pharmacological factors: the classic example of this is 'sinus arrhythmia', in which SA node activity is affected by that of the vagus nerve.

SINUS ARRHYTHMIA

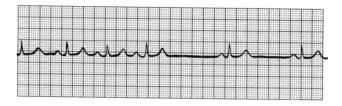

Note: Although the R–R interval varies markedly, the shape of the P waves and the duration of the PR intervals are constant. The irregularity in the rate of the QRS complexes must therefore be due to sinus arrhythmia.

Sinus arrest

Loss of SA node activity causes 'sinus arrest', a rhythm common in the sick sinus syndrome. This ECG abnormality can be differentiated from sinoatrial block because from time to time the expected P wave does not appear until after two (or three) normal intervals, and then not at the expected time.

SINUS ARREST

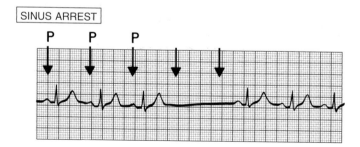

Note: Sinus rhythm
After three beats there is a 'sinus pause' with no P wave
Arrows mark where the next two P waves should have been
Sinus rhythm is then restored, but the cycle has been reset.

Escape beats

The automaticity of any part of the heart is suppressed by the arrival of a depolarization wave, and the heart rate is therefore controlled by the region with the highest automatic depolarization frequency. Normally the SA node controls the heart rate because it has the highest frequency of discharge, but if for any reason this fails the region with the next highest intrinsic depolarization frequency will emerge as the pacemaker and set up an 'escape' rhythm. The atria and the junctional region have automatic depolarization frequencies of about 50 per minute, compared with the normal SA node frequency of 60–70 per minute. If both the SA node and the junctional region fail to depolarize, or if conduction to the ventricles fails, a ventricular focus may emerge with a rate of 30–40 per minute; this is classically seen in complete heart block.

Escape beats may be single or may form sustained rhythms. They have the same ECG appearance as the corresponding extrasystoles, but appear late rather than early.

JUNCTIONAL ESCAPE BEAT

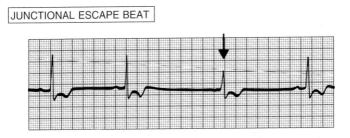

Note: After two sinus beats there is no P wave
After an interval there is a narrow QRS complex, with the same configuration as that of the sinus beats but without a preceding P wave. This is a junctional beat. Sinus rhythm then reappears.

In sustained junctional escape rhythms, atrial activation may be seen as a P wave following the QRS complex: this occurs if depolarization spreads in the opposite direction from normal, from the AV node to the atria. This is called 'retrograde' conduction.

JUNCTIONAL (ESCAPE) RHYTHM

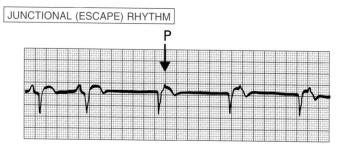

Note: Two sinus beats are followed by an interval with no P
waves
A junctional rhythm then emerges (with QRS complexes
the same as in sinus rhythm)
A P wave (arrowed) can be seen as a hump on the T wave
of the junctional beats: the atria have been depolarized
retrogradely.

JUNCTIONAL (ESCAPE) RHYTHM

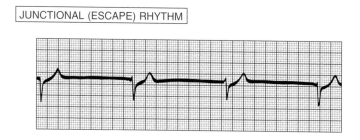

Note: No P waves
Narrow QRS complexes and normal T waves.

VENTRICULAR ESCAPE BEAT

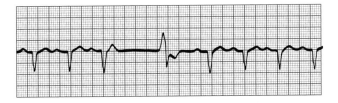

Note: Three sinus beats are followed by a pause. There is then a single ventricular beat with a wide QRS complex and an inverted T wave. Sinus rhythm is then restored.

Enhanced automaticity

If the intrinsic frequency of depolarization of the atrial, junctional or ventricular conducting tissue is increased, an abnormal rhythm may occur: this phenomenon is called 'enhanced automaticity'. The most common example of a sustained rhythm due to enhanced automaticity is 'accelerated idioventricular rhythm', which is common after acute myocardial infarction. The ECG appearance resembles a slow ventricular tachycardia, and this is the old-fashioned name for this condition. This rhythm causes no symptoms, and should not be treated.

ACCELERATED IDIOVENTRICULAR RHYTHM

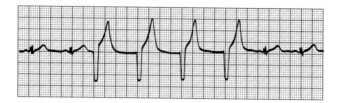

Note: After two sinus beats, there are four beats of ventricular origin with a rate of 75 per minute. Sinus rhythm is then restored.

An accelerated idionodal rhythm may appear to 'overtake' P waves if the junctional intrinsic frequency is enhanced to a point at which it approximates to that of the SA node. This rhythm used to be called a 'wandering pacemaker'.

ACCELERATED IDIONODAL RHYTHM

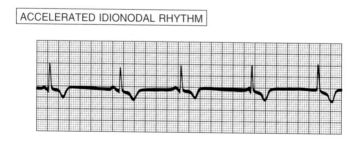

Note: After three sinus beats the sinus rate slows slightly. A nodal rhythm appears and 'overtakes' the P waves.

Enhanced automaticity is thought to be the mechanism causing some non-paroxysmal tachycardias, particularly those due to digitalis intoxication.

ABNORMALITIES OF CARDIAC RHYTHM DUE TO RE-ENTRY

Normal conduction results in the uniform spread of the depolarization wave-front in a constant direction. Should the direction of depolarization be reversed in some part of the heart, it beomes possible for a circular or 're-entry' pathway to be set up, round which depolarization reverberates, causing a tachycardia. The anatomical requirement for this is the branching and rejoining of a conduction pathway. Normally, conduction is anterograde (forward) in both limbs of such a pathway, but an anterograde impulse may pass normally down one and be blocked in the other. From the point at which the pathways rejoin, the depolarization wave can spread retrogradely (backwards) up the abnormal branch. If it arrives when that pathway is not refractory to conduction it can then pass right around the circuit and reactivate it. Once established, this circular wave of depolarization may continue until some part of the pathway fails to conduct. The conduction of a depolarization wave round a circular pathway may also be interrupted by the arrival of another depolarization wave, set up by an ectopic focus (i.e. an extrasystole).

RE-ENTRY MECHANISM CAUSING TACHYCARDIAS

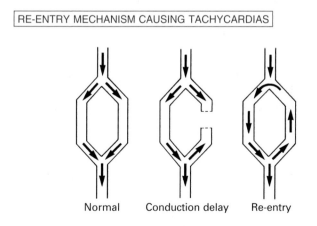

Normal　　　Conduction delay　　　Re-entry

Atrioventricular re-entry (AVRE) tachycardia

The classical, though not the most common, example of re-entry occurs in the Wolff-Parkinson-White (WPW) syndrome (see Ch. 2). Here the re-entry circuit comprises the normal AV node-His bundle connection between the atria and the ventricles, and the accessory pathway that connects the atrial muscle to the ventricular muscle on either the right or left side of the heart without involving the AV node. Depolarization can pass down the normal pathway and back up (i.e. retrogradely) through the accessory pathway to reactivate the atrium: this is called an 'orthodromic reciprocating tachycardia' and it causes narrow QRS complexes with P waves visible just after each QRS complex. Alternatively, depolarization can pass down the accessory pathway and retrogradely up the His bundle system to cause an 'antidromic reciprocating tachycardia', in which the QRS complexes are broad and slurred, and P waves may or may not be seen.

The Lown-Ganong-Levine (LGL) syndrome is due to an AV node bypass that connects the atrium to the His bundle. When re-entry occurs the QRS complexes remain narrow, with appearances similar to those of the orthodromic recriprocating tachycardia of the WPW syndrome. The tachycardias due to the WPW and LGL syndromes are grouped together under the term 'atrioventricular re-entry (AVRE) tachycardias'.

Atrial flutter

Atrial flutter is an organized atrial tachycardia due to re-entry through a small circuit within the atrial muscle.

ATRIAL FLUTTER WITH CAROTID SINUS PRESSURE (CSP)

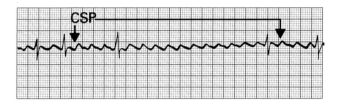

Note: Atrial flutter with 2:1 block. Carotid sinus pressure completely suppresses AV conduction, and there is no QRS complex for 3 seconds.

Atrial fibrillation

In atrial fibrillation, 'flutter-like' waves sometimes appear intermittently and these depend on re-entry through circuits of varying lengths. 'Flutter-fibrillation' behaves clinically like atrial fibrillation.

ATRIAL FIBRILLATION

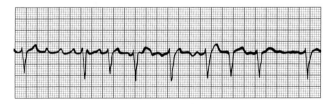

Note: Atrial fibrillation with a varying QRS complex rate but constant QRS complex configuration. Initially, 'flutter' waves are present, but later these are replaced by the typical chaotic baseline of fibrillation. This record is from V_1, which often shows atrial activity best in cases of atrial fibrillation and flutter.

Junctional tachycardia

Junctional tachycardia occurs because of a congenital abnormality of the AV node, which allows re-entry to start and be sustained within the node itself. Atrial and ventricular activation are virtually simultaneous, so the P waves are hidden within the QRS complex.

AV NODAL RE-ENTRY (JUNCTIONAL) TACHYCARDIA

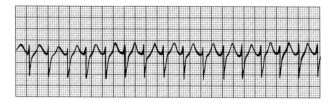

Note: No P waves can be seen. The QRS complexes are narrow and completely regular at 160 per minute.

Junctional tachycardia is the most common form of paroxysmal tachycardia in young and middle-aged people, and it is often referred to as 'supraventricular tachycardia' or 'SVT'. In fact it is only one of the supraventricular tachycardias – properly speaking, sinus tachycardia, atrial tachycardia, atrial flutter and atrial fibrillation are all types of supraventricular tachycardia.

Since the AVRE tachycardias of the WPW and LGL syndromes involve the junctional region (that is, the AV node and surrounding tissue), junctional tachycardias are most accurately called 'AV nodal re-entry' (AVNRE) tachycardias. However the terms 'junctional tachycardia' and 'SVT' seem likely to persist in common usage.

Atrial tachycardia

True atrial tachycardia is the least common of the paroxysmal narrow complex (i.e. narrow QRS complex) tachycardias. The arrhythmia arises in the atrial muscle, and the position and shape of the P wave depend on the proximity of the origin of the arrhythmia to the AV node. In some cases the arrhythmia may be due to a small re-entry circuit, but in others it may result from enhanced automaticity.

Broad complex tachycardias

If a tachycardia shows a broad QRS complex, there are three possible causes:

- a supraventricular tachycardia with bundle branch block: here the mechanism of the tachycardia is that of the supraventricular rhythm, but conduction into the ventricles occurs through one bundle branch only
- reciprocating tachycardia associated with the WPW syndrome
- ventricular tachycardia: here the arrhythmia may be due to re-entry through circuits within the Purkinje system, or may result from enhanced automaticity.

In ventricular tachycardia, the broad QRS complexes are of a constant configuration and are fairly regular if the re-entry pathway is constant.

VENTRICULAR TACHYCARDIA

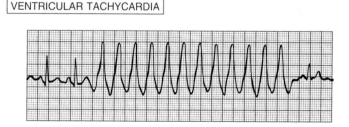

Note: Two sinus beats are followed by ventricular tachycardia at 150 per minute. The complexes are regular, with little variation in shape. Sinus rhythm is then restored.

However, the re-entry pathway often varies slightly, causing variation in the shape of the QRS complexes and some irregularity in their timing. This is seen in its most extreme form in the torsades de pointes variety of ventricular tachycardia.

VENTRICULAR TACHYCARDIA

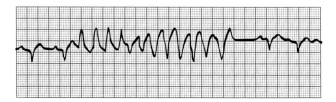

Note: Two sinus beats are followed by ventricular tachycardia. The complexes initially point upwards, but then become inverted and the QRS complex rate is variable.

DIFFERENTIATION BETWEEN RE-ENTRY AND ENHANCED AUTOMATICITY

Except in the case of the pre-excitation syndromes, there is no certain way of distinguishing from the surface ECG between a tachycardia due to enhanced automaticity and one due to re-entry. In general, however, tachycardias that follow or are terminated by extrasystoles, or those that can be initiated or inhibited by appropriately timed intracardiac pacing impulses, are likely to be due to re-entry.

ATRIAL TACHYCARDIA

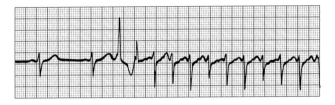

Note. After two sinus beats there is one ventricular extrasystole, and then a narrow complex which is probably supraventricular. Atrial tachycardia is induced. P waves are visible at the end of the T wave of the preceding beat.

JUNCTIONAL TACHYCARDIA

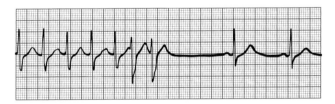

Note: Five beats of junctional tachycardia at 150 per minute are followed by two ventricular extrasystoles. These interrupt the tachycardia, and sinus rhythm is restored.

The differentiation between tachycardias caused by enhanced automaticity and those caused by re-entry does not affect the choice of treatment.

The following full ECG shows a combination of abnormalities which can be explained in physiological terms.

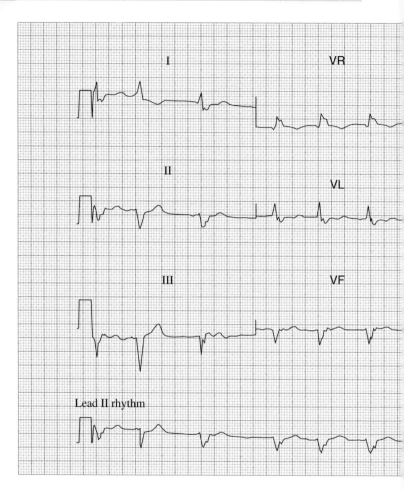

This ECG was recorded from an 84-year-old man who had complained of intermittent palpitations for many years, and who developed increasing heart failure over a period of a few months. The EGC shows:

- Atrial fibrillation, with one ventricular extrasystole (seen in leads V₄–V₆)
- Left axis deviation

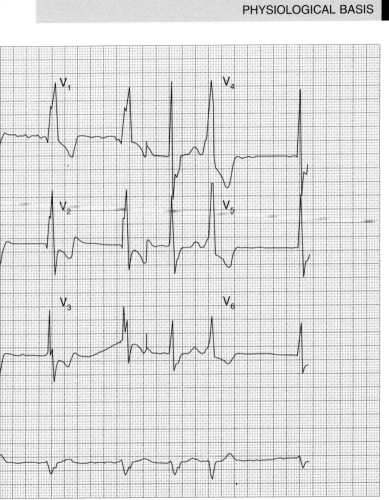

- Broad QRS complexes, with an RSR^1 pattern in V_1 and a wide S wave in V_6.

Interpretation:

Atrial fibrillation and bifascicular block. This patient had a dilated cardiomyopathy.

CHAPTER 7
Reminders

Remember that interpreting the ECG is only a small part of making a diagnosis. The following lists are to remind you of the variations in the ECG seen in normal people, of some of the possible causes of specific ECG abnormalities, and of some of the diseases that an ECG may suggest.

WHAT CAN BE ACCEPTED AS NORMAL?

Acceptable variations in the normal ECG in adults

Rhythm

Marked sinus arrhythmia, with escape beats
Lack of sinus arrhythmia (normal with increasing age)
Supraventricular extrasystoles
Ventricular extrasystoles.

P wave

Normally inverted in VR
May be inverted in VL.

Cardiac axis

Minor right axis deviation in tall people
Minor left axis deviation in fat people and in pregnancy.

QRS complexes in the chest leads

Slight dominance of R wave in V_1, provided there is no other

evidence of RV hypertrophy or posterior infarction
The R wave in the lateral chest leads may exceed 25 mm
in thin fit young people
Partial right bundle branch block (RSR_1 pattern, with QRS
complexes less than 120 ms)
Septal Q waves in III, VL, V_5–V_6.

ST segment

Raised in anterior leads following an S wave (high take-off)
Depressed in pregnancy
Nonspecific, upward sloping, depression.

T wave

Inverted in VR and often in V_1
Inverted in V_2, V_3 or even V_4 in Black people
May invert with hyperventilation
Peaked, especially if the T waves are tall.

U wave

Normal in anterior leads when the T wave is not flattened.

The ECG in normal children

At birth

Sinus tachycardia
Right axis deviation
Dominant R waves in V_1
Deep S waves in V_6
Inverted T waves in V_1–V_4.

At 1 year of age

Sinus tachycardia
Right axis deviation
Dominant R waves in V_1
Inverted T waves in V_1–V_2.

At 2 years of age

Normal axis
S waves exceed R waves in V_1
T waves inverted in V_1–V_2.

At 5 years of age

Normal QRS complexes
T waves still inverted in V_1–V_2.

At 10 years of age

Adult pattern.

Acceptable variations in the ECG in athletes

Sinus arrhythmia
"Wandering atrial pacemaker"
First degree block
Wenckebach block
Junctional rhythm
Slight elevation of ST segments
Tall, symmetrical T waves
Prominent Q waves in lateral leads
Tall R waves
Prominent U waves.

ECG in pregnancy

Sinus tachycardia
Supraventricular and ventricular extrasystoles
Nonspecific ST segment/T wave changes.

ASSOCIATIONS AND POSSIBLE CAUSES OF PARTICULAR ECG PATTERNS

The P wave

Absent P waves

Atrial fibrillation

Sinoatrial block
Hyperkalaemia
Junctional (AV nodal) rhythm, e.g. in sick sinus syndrome.

Peaked P waves

Lung disease
Pulmonary embolus
Primary pulmonary hypertension
Pulmonary or tricuspid valve stenosis.

The QRS complex

Left axis deviation

Left anterior hemiblock
Inferior wall infarction
Ventricular tachycardia from left ventricular focus
Some types of Wolff-Parkinson-White syndrome
Congenital heart disease, e.g. endocardial cushion defects,
corrected transposition.

N.B. Left ventricular hypertrophy in itself does not cause left axis
deviation; pregnancy and obesity only cause minor degrees of left
axis deviation.

*Left anterior hemiblock (conduction defect in antero-superior
division of left bundle branch)*

Intermittent
Any rapid supraventricular rhythm.

Persistent
Fibrosis associated with:
Ischaemic disease
Cardiomyopathy
Long-standing hypertension
Long-standing congestive failure of any cause.

Right axis deviation

Right ventricular hypertrophy due to any cause

Pulmonary embolus
Antero-lateral myocardial infarction
Wolff-Parkinson-White syndrome with left-sided bypass
Left posterior hemiblock (rare).

Low voltage QRS complexes

Incorrect standardization
Emphysema
Obesity
Pericardial effusion
Myxoedema
Hypopituitarism.

Wide QRS complexes

Rhythms with a ventricular origin (extrasystoles, tachycardias,
accelerated idioventricular rhythms, escape rhythms such as
complete block)
Left anterior hemiblock
Right bundle branch block
Left bundle branch block.

Right bundle branch block

Seen in normal subjects
Atrial septal defect
Pulmonary embolus
Cor pulmonale.

Left bundle branch block

Occasionally seen in healthy subjects
Ischaemic heart disease
Cardiomyopathy
Hypertension
Idiopathic fibrosis.

Q waves

Normal if less than 40 ms duration or 2 mm deep
'Septal' Q waves normal in the lateral leads
Common in normal records in III, V_5–V_6
Myocardial infarction of more than a few hours' duration.

Dominant R waves in V_1

Minor R wave dominance can be normal
Associated with right bundle branch block
Pulmonary embolus
Right ventricular hypertrophy due to any cause
Posterior myocardial infarction
Myocarditis
WPW syndrome with left-sided pathway.

The QT interval and ST segment

Long QT interval

QT interval lengthens somewhat during sleep
Congenital:
    Jervell-Lange-Nielsen syndrome (includes deafness)
    Romano-Ward syndrome (no deafness)
Acute myocarditis due to any cause
Acute myocardial infarction
Cerebral injury
Hypothermia
Complete AV block
Low serum calcium, potassium, or magnesium level
Class Ia anti-arrhythmic drugs, e.g. quinidine, procainamide
Other drugs, including tricyclic antidepressants and chloroquine.

Short QT interval

Digitalis
Hypercalcaemia
Hyperthermia.

N.B. The faster the heart rate, the shorter the QT interval.

ST segment depression

Normal if upward-sloping
Nonspecific if concave upwards and the depression is less than 2 mm
Digitalis if downsloping
Ischaemic if horizontal.

ST segment elevation

Normal variant (high take-off)
Acute myocardial infarction
Prinzmetal's angina
Pericarditis
Left ventricular aneurysm
During stress testing, may be due to impaired LV function.

The T wave

Anterior T wave inversion

In V_1–V_3 or V_4
Normal in Black people and children
Right bundle branch block
Pulmonary embolism.

In V_2–V_5
Non-Q wave myocardial infarction
Hypertrophic cardiomyopathy
Subarachnoid haemorrhage
Lithium treatment

In V_4–V_6
Left ventricular hypertrophy
Ischaemia
Associated with left bundle branch block.

Lateral T wave inversion

Ischaemia

Left ventricular hypertrophy
Associated with left bundle branch block.

Flattening of the T wave

Pericardial effusion
Hypokalaemia
Hypothyroidism.

The U wave

May be normal
Hypokalaemia
Hypocalcaemia
Hypothyroidism.

Tachycardias and bradycardias

Slow rhythms

Sinus bradycardia
Sick sinus syndrome
Second or third degree block
Escape rhythms
Drugs.

Narrow complex tachycardias

The effect of carotid sinus pressure is shown in parentheses:
Sinus (slows)
Atrial (arrhythmia abolished or no effect)
Atrioventricular re-entry (junctional) (arrhythmia abolished or no effect)
Atrial flutter (increased AV block)
Atrial fibrillation (no effect).

Broad complex tachycardias

Supraventricular rhythm with bundle branch block
Ventricular tachycardia

Accelerated idioventricular rhythm (rate less than 120 per min)
Torsades de pointes.

Broad complex tachycardias are usually ventricular in the
context of acute myocardial infarction.

Differentiation of broad complex tachycardias

Comparison with record taken in sinus rhythm
Identification of P waves (independent P waves in ventricular
tachycardia)
QRS complex width: if greater than 160 ms, usually ventricular
QRS complex regularity: if very irregular, probably AF with
conduction defect
Cardiac axis: left axis deviation, especially with right bundle
branch block, is usually ventricular
Any axis change compared with sinus rhythm probably indicates
ventricular origin.

Concordance
VT is likely if the QRS complex is predominantly upward, or
predominantly downward, in all the chest leads.

With right bundle branch block pattern:
Ventricular origin is likely if:
Left axis deviation
Tall R waves in V_1
R taller than R^1 in V_1

With left bundle branch block pattern:
Ventricular origin is likely if:
QS wave (i.e. no R wave) in V_6.

Capture beats
Narrow complex following short R–R interval (i.e. an early narrow
beat interrupting a broad complex tachycardia) suggests that basic
rhythm is ventricular.

Fusion beats
An intermediate QRS complex pattern arises when the ventricles

are activated simultaneously by a supraventricular and a ventricular impulse.

Sick sinus syndrome variants

Inappropriate sinus bradycardia
Sinoatrial arrest
Sinus node exit block
'Silent atrium' – junctional escape
Bradycardia-tachycardia syndrome
Atrial fibrillation with slow ventricular response.

The ECG and the peripheral pulse

Rhythms that may underlie an apparently normal or slightly slow pulse rate

Sinus bradycardia
Atrial flutter with 3:1 or 4:1 block
Second degree (2:1) block
Complete AV block with a ventricular escape rate of about 50 per minute
Sick sinus syndrome with idionodal rhythm
Idioventricular rhythm.

Rhythms that may underlie an irregular pulse

Marked sinus arrhythmia
Supraventricular or ventricular extrasystoles
Atrial fibrillation
Flutter with variable block
Varying sinus rhythm and AV block.

ECG PATTERNS WHICH MAY BE ASSOCIATED WITH SPECIFIC CONDITIONS

Congenital heart disease

Pulmonary stenosis

Right atrial and right ventricular hypertrophy.

Fallot's tetralogy

Right atrial and right ventricular hypertrophy.

Atrial septal defect

Left atrial or right atrial hypertrophy
Partial or complete right bundle branch block.

Ventricular septal defect

Normal
Left ventricular hypertrophy.

Eisenmenger's syndrome

Right ventricular hypertrophy.

Valve disease

Mitral stenosis

Atrial fibrillation
Left atrial hypertrophy, if in sinus rhythm
Right ventricular hypertrophy.

Mitral regurgitation

Atrial fibrillation
Left atrial hypertrophy, if in sinus rhythm
Left ventricular hypertrophy.

Aortic stenosis

Left ventricular hypertrophy
Incomplete left bundle branch block (i.e. loss of Q waves in V_5–V_6)
Left bundle branch block.

Aortic regurgitation

Left ventricular hypertrophy

Prominent but narrow Q wave in V_6
Left anterior hemiblock
Occasionally, left bundle branch block.

Mitral valve prolapse

Sinus rhythm, or wide variety of arrhythmias
Inverted T waves in II, III and VF
T wave inversion in precordial leads
ST segment depression
Exercise-induced ventricular arrhythmias.

N.B. Abnormalities can vary in different records from the same individual.

Biventricular hypertrophy

Left ventricular hypertrophy plus right axis deviation
Left ventricular hypertrophy plus clockwise rotation
Left ventricular hypertrophy with tall R waves in V_1.

Congestive cardiomyopathy

Arrhythmias, especially atrial fibrillation and ventricular tachycardia
First degree block
Right or left atrial enlargement
Low amplitude QRS complexes
Left anterior hemiblock
Left bundle branch block
Right bundle branch block
Left ventricular hypertrophy
Nonspecific ST segment and T wave changes.

Hypertrophic cardiomyopathy

Short PR interval
Various rhythm disturbances, including ventricular tachycardia, ventricular fibrillation
Left atrial hypertrophy

Left anterior hemiblock or left bundle branch block
Left ventricular hypertrophy
Prolonged QT interval
Deep T wave inversion anteriorly.

Myocarditis

Sinus tachycardias and other arrhythmias
First, second or third degree block
Widened QRS complexes
Irregularity of QRS wave-form
Q waves
Prolonged QT interval
ST segment elevation or depression
T wave inversion in any lead.

Acute rheumatic fever

Sinus tachycardia
First degree block
Changes of acute myocarditis
Changes associated with pericarditis.

Pulmonary embolism

Sinus tachycardia
Atrial arrhythmias
Right atrial hypertrophy
Right ventricular hypertrophy
Right axis deviation
Clockwise rotation with persistent S wave in V_6
Right bundle branch block
Combination of S wave in lead I with Q wave and inverted T wave in lead III.

Chronic obstructive pulmonary disease

Small complexes
Right atrial hypertrophy (P pulmonale)

Right axis deviation
Right ventricular hypertrophy
Clockwise rotation (deep S waves in V_6)
Right bundle branch block.

Potassium and magnesium imbalance

Low:
Flattened T waves
U waves
First or second degree block
Depressed ST segments.

High:
Flat or absent P waves
Widening of QRS complexes
Intraventricular conduction delay
Tall, wide, peaked, symmetrical T waves
Disappearance of ST segment
Arrhythmias.

Calcium imbalance

Low:
Prolonged QT interval, due to prolonged ST segment.

High:
Short QT interval, with absent ST segment.

Digitalis

Downsloping ST segments
Flattened or inverted T waves
Short QT interval
Almost any abnormal cardiac rhythm, but especially:
Sinus bradycardia
Paroxysmal atrial tachycardia with AV block
Ventricular extrasystoles

Ventricular tachycardia
Any degree of AV block
Regularization of QRS complexes in atrial fibrillation suggests toxicity.

Wolff-Parkinson-White syndrome

Short PR interval
Slight widening of QRS complexes: delta wave with normal terminal segment
ST segment/T wave changes
Arrhythmias (narrow or wide complex)
Arrhythmia with wide, irregular complex suggests WPW syndrome with AF
Right-sided pathway: sometimes, anterior T wave inversion
Left-sided pathway: dominant R waves in V_1–V_6.

Exercise testing

Stress testing may reveal:
Patient's attitude to exercise
Reason for exercise intolerance (breathlessness etc.)
Ventricular performance: heart rate and blood pressure response
Ischaemia
Exercise-induced arrhythmias.

The ECG recorded during exercise testing is unreliable in cases of:
Bundle branch block
Ventricular hypertrophy
Wolff-Parkinson-White syndrome
Digoxin therapy
Beta-blocker therapy.

POSSIBLE CAUSES OF ECG ABNORMALITIES

Remember that there are several clinical causes of all ECG abnormalities: there is always a differential diagnosis.

Sinus tachycardia

Pain, fright, exercise
Hypovolaemia
Myocardial infarction
Heart failure
Pulmonary embolism
Obesity
Lack of physical fitness
Pregnancy
Thyrotoxicosis
Anaemia
Beri-beri
CO_2 retention
Autonomic neuropathy
Drugs:
  Sympathomimetics
  Salbutamol (including by inhalation)
  Caffeine
  Atropine.

Sinus bradycardia

Physical fitness
Vaso-vagal attacks
Sick sinus syndrome
Acute myocardial infarction, especially inferior
Hypothyroidism
Hypothermia
Obstructive jaundice
Raised intracranial pressure
Drugs:
  Beta-blockers (including eye-drops for glaucoma)
  Verapamil
  Digoxin.

Sick sinus syndrome

Familial:
  Isolated

With atrioventricular conduction disturbance
With QT interval prolongation
Congenital
Acquired:
    Idiopathic
    Coronary disease
    Rheumatic disease
    Cardiomyopathy
    Neuromuscular disease:
        Friedreich's ataxia
        Peroneal muscular atrophy
        Charcot-Marie-Tooth disease
    Infiltration:
        Amyloidosis
        Haemochromatosis
    Collagen diseases:
        Rheumatoid
        Scleroderma
        SLE
    Myocarditis:
        Viral
        Diphtheria
    Drugs:
        Lithium
        Aerosol propellants.

Atrial fibrillation (paroxysmal or persistent)

Rheumatic heart disease
Thyrotoxicosis
Alcoholism
Cardiomyopathy
Acute myocardial infarction
Chronic ischaemic heart disease
Hypertension
Myocarditis
Pericarditis
Pulmonary embolism
Pneumonia

Cardiac surgery
Wolff-Parkinson-White syndrome
'Lone'.

Ventricular tachycardia

Acute myocardial infarction
Chronic ischaemia
Cardiomyopathy:
    Hypertrophic
    Dilated
Mitral valve prolapse
Myocarditis
Electrolyte imbalance
Congenital long QT syndrome
Drugs:
    Anti-arrhythmic
    Digoxin
Idiopathic.

Torsades de pointes ventricular tachycardia

Class I anti-arrhythmic drugs
Amiodarone
Sotalol
Tricyclic antidepressants.

Electromechanical dissociation (EMD arrest)

Tamponade
Drug overdose
Electrolyte imbalance
Hypothermia
Pulmonary embolism
Tension pneumothorax.

Heart block

First and second degree

Normal variant

Increased vagal tone
Athletes
Sick sinus syndrome
Acute carditis
Ischaemic disease
Hypokalaemia
Lyme disease (*Borrelia burgdorferi*)
Digoxin
Beta-blockers
Calcium-channel blockers.

Complete block

Idiopathic (conduction tissue fibrosis)
Congenital
Ischaemic disease
Associated with aortic valve calcification
Cardiac surgery and trauma
Digitalis intoxication
Bundle interruption by tumours, parasites, abscesses,
granulomas, injury.

Pericarditis

Viral
Bacterial (including TB)
Dressler's syndrome post myocardial infarction
Malignancy
Uraemia
Acute rheumatic fever
Myxoedema
Connective tissue diseases
Radiotherapy.

Myocarditis

Viral

Coxsackie B3
Hepatitis

Mumps
Influenza.

Bacterial

Septicaemia
Tuberculosis.

Rickettsial

Scrub typhus.

Mycotic

Histoplasmosis
Actinomycosis.

Parasitic

Chagas' disease.

Prolapsing mitral valve syndrome

Primary degeneration of chordae
Coronary disease and papillary muscle dysfunction
Acute carditis
Marfan's syndrome
Hypertrophic cardiomyopathy
Wolff-Parkinson-White syndrome
Hereditary long QT syndromes.

Hypokalaemia

Diuretic therapy
Antidiuretic hormone secretion.

Hyperkalaemia

Renal failure

Potassium-retaining diuretics (amiloride, spironolactone, triamterine)
Angiotensin-converting enzyme inhibitors
Liquorice
Bartter's syndrome.

Hypocalcaemia

Hypoparathyroidism
Severe diarrhoea
Enteric fistulae
Alkalosis
Vitamin D deficiency.

Hypercalcaemia

Hyperparathyroidism
Renal failure
Sarcoidosis
Malignancy
Myeloma
Excess vitamin D
Thiazide diuretics.

Conclusions

The ECG is basically easy to understand, and most of its abnormalities are perfectly logical. As in everything in biology and medicine, there are quite marked variations – in both the ECGs of normal subjects and the ECG patterns that accompany specific diseases – and it is these variations that sometimes make ECG interpretation seem difficult. These variations will be recognized with practice and as a learning mechanism there is no substitute for reporting large numbers of ECGs, whether these be normal or abnormal.

However, the key to the ECG is to use it as an adjunct to the patient's history and physical examination. When in doubt, it is better to depend on these than on the ECG and it is always the patient who should be treated, not the ECG.

Now test yourself: *100 ECG Problems*, a companion to this volume, gives 100 clinical scenarios with full ECGs, and poses questions about ECG interpretation and patient management.

Index

Your COMPLETE Guide to the ECG

The ECG Made Easy

John R Hampton

July 1997   0 443 05681 1
International Edition available: 0443 05695 1

This popular text provides a readable guide to ECG interpretation, with an emphasis throughout on straightforward practical application. Whatever your clinical role, make sure you have the ideal pocket reference to this essential diagnostic tool!

"ideal for students wishing to learn the basic essentials of electrocardiography ... good value for money."

Mediscope

"a godsend to thousands of practising physicians and surgeons who never really mastered the ECG but always felt that they should have done."

European Medical Journal

The ECG in Practice
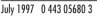

John R Hampton

July 1997   0 443 05680 3

Although the ECG is easy in principle, variations in its pattern can make it seem complex. **The ECG in Practice** is a companion volume to **The ECG Made Easy**. It has been written to help you make the most of the ECG – and to appreciate its limitations.

"*the* pocket reference for junior doctors."

Nursing Standard

"an excellent book for medical students and junior medical staff."

Cardiovascular Research

100 ECG Problems

John R Hampton

July 1997   0 443 05678 1

There is no substitute for reporting a large number of ECGs. This book provides 100 real clinical case histories, with the 12-lead ECG from each patient. You are asked to report and interpret each ECG, and to draw up a plan for the patient's management. The answers are given on the reverse of the page showing the ECG.